THE FAMILY GUIDE TO

Prescription Drugs

Compiled and reviewed by:

THE PHARMEX
PROFESSIONAL REVIEW COMMITTEE

J. Richard Wuest, R.Ph., Pharm. D.

Thomas A. Gossel, R.Ph., Ph.D.

Henry A. Palmer, R.Ph., Ph.D.

Nicholas G. Popovich, R.Ph., Ph.D.

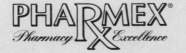

Published by

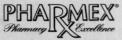

PHARMEX®
Pharmacy R *Excellence*

A division of Automatic Business Products, Co., Inc.

1531 Airway Circle, New Smyrna Beach, FL 32168

IMPORTANT

THE FAMILY GUIDE TO PRESCRIPTION DRUGS has been designed to provide general information only and is not a substitute for professional judgement or advice given in individual cases. The contents of the monographs are not intended to take the place of specific directions the patient may have received from his or her physician, pharmacist or health care professional. And such professionals should be consulted should the patient suffer from allergies or have any questions about the drug being taken.

The authors and publishers of this material cannot be responsible for errors or any other consequences arising from its use.

First Printing, September ,1980
Second Printing, February, 1981
Third Printing, July, 1993

Contents Printed in the U.S.A.

TABLE OF CONTENTS

PREFACE

The Family Guide to Prescription Drugs will give you important information about your medications in understandable language. It will tell you what the medicine is used for, how to take it properly, what significant side effects to watch for, as well as other meaningful facts about the prescription drugs you are taking.

The beginning of the Guide (pages 1-12) contains instructions on the proper use of various forms of medicines such as eye drops and ear drops. The remainder of this Guide contains information on particular drugs. There is an index in the back to help you locate information on specific drugs.

 The Pharmex Professional Review Committee, with years of professional and academic experience in providing drug information, has examined the information on each drug for accuracy.

 Pharmex originated the idea of providing attention getting graphics on warning labels and manufactures most of the warning labels you see on prescription containers. Pharmex also invented and patented the first multiple roll warning label dispenser. This dispenser was recognized by the Smithsonian Institute as being the "state of the art" in pharmacy practice.

 Pharmex has been a leader in compiling drug information leaflets that have been provided to patients by pharmacists and other health care professionals for nearly 20 years.

FOREWORD

As shown by the statistics printed on the back cover of this Guide, the efforts of health care professionals are often blocked by patients who don't take their medicines as prescribed. Taking a medicine properly is as important as taking the proper medicine.

To help patients be better informed, the National Council on Patient Information and Education (NCPIE) suggests that consumers get answers to five important questions about their medications.

1. What is the name of the medicine and what is it supposed to do?

 2. How and when do I take it and for how long?

 3. What foods, drinks, other medicines or activities should I avoid while taking this medicine?

 4. Are there any significant side effects and what should I do if they occur?

 5. Is there any written information available about the medicine?

This Guide will be very helpful in providing you with this type of information. Let's review each of these questions.

 1. What is the name of the medicine and what it is supposed to do? Many medications are sold under several different brand names and a generic name. Since some patients see more than one doctor, it is possible that one doctor might prescribe the same (or similar) medication as another doctor, not being aware that the patient is already taking the medication. If the drug is sold under two different names and the patient is not aware of it, the dosage can be unintentionally duplicated. This is why it is helpful to show each doctor all the medications you are taking. Also, if you buy all your medicine at one pharmacy, the pharmacist will know all the medications you are taking and be able to spot these duplications. Most importantly, you should know what each of your medicines is and what they were prescribed for.

2. How and when do I take it and for how long? How to take a medicine is very important. Some liquids are intended to be swallowed and some rubbed on the skin or placed in the ear or eye. Although most tablets and capsules are obviously intended to be swallowed, some tablet-like medicines should be inserted rectally or vaginally. There have been instances where an antibiotic liquid is prescribed for a child with an earache and the liquid, which was supposed to be swallowed, is placed into the child's ear.

Sometimes, simple directions like "twice a day" are confusing. Does this mean the doses should be taken exactly twelve hours apart, or in the morning and afternoon? When the prescriber gives the instructions "take every four hours," does that mean around the clock or just while awake? Since there are no standard answers to these types of questions, it is important to check with your doctor or pharmacist.

How long to continue taking the medicine also depends on the situation. Some drugs, such as most antibiotics, should be taken for 7-10 days for the treatment to be effective. In this case, even if the patient is feeling better after a few days, discontinuing the medication may cause the illness to return. Medicines which are used to relieve symptoms, such as many cough remedies, often need to be taken only when the symptom is present. Others are used to control a condition, such as high blood pressure, and should always be taken, even when you are feeling well. There are many exceptions to this and, as always, if you have any questions, check with your health care professional.

 3. What foods, drinks, other medicines or activities should I avoid while taking this medicine? Some medicines work better when taken with food while others should be taken without food. You should find out before taking the medicine which way is best.

Of course, alcoholic beverages can have undesirable effects when taken with some prescription (and non-prescription) drugs. This may include increased dizziness or drowsiness. Other drinks, such as colas and even milk, can also conflict with the action of medicines. It is normally best to take tablets and capsules with a full glass of water.

Some drugs can have adverse reactions to each other. Here again, it is useful to purchase all of your prescriptions in the same pharmacy and inform your doctor of all the medicines you are taking. Your doctor or pharmacist can then tell if you are taking medicines which may interact with each other. This applies to non-prescription medications as well.

As far as activities to avoid, we are often reminded to not drive a car or operate dangerous machinery while taking medications that may make us drowsy or dizzy. However other activities, such as exercise, can change a medicine's effectiveness. You should ask your doctor to review your lifestyle to determine if there are activities you should avoid.

 4. Are there any significant side effects and what do I do if they occur? The potential for side effects should not discourage an individual from taking the prescribed medicine. Presumably, the prescriber has weighed any potential negative reactions the drug may have against the drug's benefits. Also, it is important that if you do suffer from side effects that you inform your doctor or pharmacist, especially before taking non-prescription remedies to counteract the side effect. For instance, if a drug causes indigestion, taking an antacid to relieve the stomach may interfere with the performance of other drugs you are taking.

 5. Is there any written information available about the medicine? In addition to the concise material contained in this Guide, you can also ask your doctor or pharmacist for additional printed material on particular drugs.

Keeping these points in mind, as well as using this Guide as a reference, will help you to be a well-informed patient and an active member of your health care team.

GENERAL INSTRUCTIONS FOR THE SAFE USE OF YOUR MEDICINE

Be sure your doctor and pharmacist know about any allergies you have to drugs (both prescription and non-prescription).

Tell your doctor if you are pregnant, plan to become pregnant or are breastfeeding.

Store your medication in a cool, dry place.

DO NOT keep medications in your bathroom medicine cabinet or in an area with excessive heat or cold.

NEVER use medications after the expiration date on the label. Ask your pharmacist if you have any questions about this.

When you have a prescription refilled, if it is not the same size or color or has different markings than before, call your pharmacist. Generic forms of the same drug do not look alike so if your pharmacist has not explained why the medication dispensed looks different from what you received previously, it is best to check and make sure it was correctly refilled.

NEVER give your medication to others.

Call your doctor if you develop a skin rash, hives or itching, swelling of the face or difficulty in breathing. These are signs of an allergic reaction to the medication.

Most people experience few or no side effects from their medication. However, if the medicine is bothering you and causing unusual reactions, call your doctor or pharmacist.

Never change the amount of medicine taken nor stop taking it without first consulting your doctor.

Always keep your medicine in its original container with the cap on tightly.

DO NOT keep or use outdated medication. Keep all medication out of the reach of children.

In case of accidental ingestion or overdose, call your doctor or poison control center immediately.

HOW TO USE
EYE DROPS

Wash your hands with soap and water before using the eye drops.

Gently pull lower eyelid downward to form a pouch.

Tilt head backward, hold the dropper above the eye and drop the prescribed amount of medicine inside the lower lid.

DO NOT touch the dropper to any surface.

Release lower lid. Try not to blink for a few seconds. Replace the cap on the bottle.

NEVER rinse the dropper. You may contaminate the medication.

Eye drops may blur your vision for a few minutes. If they do, DO NOT drive or perform hazardous tasks until your vision has cleared.

NEVER use eye drops that have changed color or appear to have crystals in the solution.

Call your doctor if your condition becomes worse or if you experience itching or burning for more than a few minutes after placing drops in the eye.

If you are using more than 1 kind of eye drop at the same time, wait at least 5 minutes before you use another eye drop. Check with your doctor or pharmacist about which one to use first.

If you wear contact lenses, remove them before instilling the eye drops.

DO NOT keep or use outdated medication. Keep all medication out of the reach of children.

In case of accidental ingestion, call your doctor or poison control center immediately.

HOW TO USE
EYE OINTMENTS

 Wash your hands with soap and water before using the eye ointment.

Gently pull lower eyelid downward to form a pouch.

 Looking in a mirror, carefully apply a small amount of ointment (about one-fourth inch) inside the lower lid.

DO NOT touch tip of tube to any surface.

Release lower lid and wipe off any ointment that may have gotten on your skin.

Replace the cap on the tube.

 Eye ointments often cause blurring of vision for a short time. DO NOT drive or perform hazardous tasks until your vision has cleared.

 Call your doctor if your condition becomes worse or if you experience itching or burning for more than a few minutes after placing in the eye.

If you are using more than 1 kind of eye ointment at the same time, wait about 5 minutes before you use another eye ointment. Check with your doctor or pharmacist about which one to use first.

 If you are using both an eye drop and an eye ointment: Instill the eye drop first, wait at least 5 minutes and apply the eye ointment.

Keep container tightly closed when not in use.

If you wear contact lenses, remove them before applying the eye ointment.

DO NOT keep or use outdated medication. Keep all medication out of the reach of children.

 In case of accidental ingestion, call your doctor or poison control center immediately.

HOW TO USE
NOSE DROPS AND SPRAYS

HOW TO USE NASAL SPRAYS:

If this product is a metered pump, it must be primed several times when first opened.

Blow your nose gently just before using.

Wash your hands with soap and water before and after using the nasal spray.

 DO NOT shake the plastic squeeze or pump bottle unless instructed to do so.

Hold head upright to spray.

 Remove the protective cap and insert nosepiece into one nostril pointing it slightly inward.

Administer the prescribed dosage as directed on the bottle, inhaling as you are squeezing or using the pump.

Wipe the applicator nozzle and repeat in other nostril.

After use, rinse the nasal tip with hot water, wipe it clean and replace the protective cap.

HOW TO USE NOSE DROPS:

Blow your nose gently before using.

Squeeze the rubber bulb to draw up 2-3 drops of medication.

Sit in a chair with head tilted back.

 Insert the dropper into one nostril and squeeze the medication into the nose. Repeat in the other nostril.

Then lean your head forward toward your knees. Inhale and hold there for a few seconds.

Be extra careful not to touch the side of the dropper to the inside of the nose or any other surface.

 After use, rinse the dropper with hot water, wipe it clean and carefully replace in bottle.

SPECIAL INSTRUCTIONS:

DO NOT use nasal solutions that have become discolored or have changed appearance.

Use of the dropper or spray unit by more than one person may spread infection.

 Call your doctor if your condition becomes worse or if you experience stinging, drying or burning of the nostrils.

Keep container tightly closed when not in use.

DO NOT keep or use outdated medication. Keep all medication out of the reach of children.

In case of accidental ingestion, call your doctor or poison control center immediately.

HOW TO USE
EAR DROPS

 Wash your hands with soap and water before and after using the ear drops.

Avoid touching the dropper against the ear or any other surface. For accuracy and to avoid contamination, another person should insert the ear drops when possible.

 Tilt head sideways with ear to be treated facing upward.

Place the prescribed dosage as instructed on the bottle into the ear.

Avoid touching the dropper to the ear.

Keep drops in the ear for several minutes by keeping head tilted or placing cotton in the ear.

Repeat in other ear if instructed to do so.

Keep container tightly closed when not in use.

 Call your doctor if your condition persists or becomes worse or if you experience itching or burning in your ear for more than a few minutes after placing the drops in the ear.

 DO NOT refrigerate, unless instructed to do so by your doctor or pharmacist.

DO NOT use any ear drop that has discolored or change in appearance.

IMPORTANT:

 DO NOT keep or use outdated medication. Keep all medication out of the reach of children.

In case of accidental ingestion, call your doctor or poison control center immediately.

HOW TO USE
ORAL INHALERS

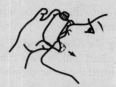

BE SURE the canister is properly inserted into the inhaler unit.

 REMOVE dust cap and SHAKE the can WELL.

Hold the inhaler with the nozzle down.

Unless your doctor has told you otherwise, exhale fully and place mouthpiece into your mouth with your lips closed around it and your tongue flat.

As you take a deep breath, squeeze the can and mouthpiece together at exactly the same time.

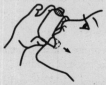

Continue taking a deep breath and hold it for as long as comfortable.

Exhale slowly keeping your lips nearly closed.

Desired relief may not be immediate. Be sure to wait the prescribed time before inhaling a second dose.

Notify your doctor if shortness of breath persists after the dose, or, if the dose fails to provide the usual relief.

KEEP THE MOUTHPIECE CLEAN. At least once daily, wash the mouthpiece with soap and hot water. Rinse thoroughly and allow to dry.

Instructions for each brand of inhaler are similar, but slightly different. Read them carefully and follow the directions. If you have any questions, ask your doctor or pharmacist.

The contents of the can are under pressure. DO NOT puncture or throw it into an incinerator.

When not using the inhaler, store it with the dust cap on the mouthpiece. This will prevent dirt and dust from getting into the mouthpiece.

DO NOT keep or use outdated medicine. Keep this medicine at room temperature, in its original container and out of the reach of children.

In case of accidental overdose, call your doctor or poison control center immediately.

HOW TO USE VAGINAL PREPARATIONS

HOW TO USE VAGINAL CREAMS:

 Wash your hands with soap and water before and after using this medication.

Read any directions for use provided by the manufacturer.

To open the tube, puncture the tube with point of cap. Screw applicator onto the tube.

 Squeeze the tube from the bottom until the plunger is extended to the appropriate mark for prescribed dose.

 Unscrew the filled applicator from the tube and insert the barrel gently into the vagina with a downward motion as far as it will comfortably go.

 This is easiest if you are lying on your back with your legs spread apart and knees bent.

Push the plunger all the way to deposit the cream into the vagina. With the plunger still pressed remove the applicator.

Pull the applicator apart for easy cleaning.

Wash the two parts with soap and lukewarm water, then dry.

DO NOT boil or soak in very hot water.

Reassemble by gently pushing the plunger back into the barrel as far as it will go.

Place cap on tube and close tightly.

HOW TO USE VAGINAL SUPPOSITORIES AND TABLETS:

 Wash your hands with soap and water before and after using this medication.

Cleanse the vaginal area and pat dry.

Remove the wrapper from the suppository/tablet.

Moisten the suppository/tablet with warm water.

 If an applicator is used, place the small end of the suppository/tablet into the applicator.

 Lie on your back with knees bent and slightly spread apart. Insert the barrel, containing the medication, gently into the vagina with a downward motion as far as it will comfortably go.

 Press the plunger gently to deposit the suppository/tablet into the vagina. With the plunger still pressed remove the applicator.

Pull the applicator apart for easy cleaning.

Wash the two parts with soap and lukewarm water, then dry.

DO NOT boil or soak in very hot water.

Reassemble by gently pushing the plunger back into the barrel as far as it will go.

SPECIAL INSTRUCTIONS:

It is recommended that you use a sanitary napkin to prevent staining of clothing.

Use continuously, even through your menstrual period.

If you experience vaginal burning or itching which was not present prior to your use of the medication or if your condition becomes worse, contact your doctor.

DO NOT keep or use outdated medication. Keep all medication out of the reach of children.

 In case of accidental ingestion, call your doctor or poison control center immediately.

HOW TO USE
TOPICAL PREPARATIONS

This product is for EXTERNAL USE ONLY.

 Wash your hands before and after using this medicine.

Cleanse the skin area with soap and water and pat dry each time you are ready to apply the medicine, unless otherwise directed by your doctor.

 Apply a small amount of the medication to the affected area and spread lightly.

Only the medicine that is actually touching the skin will work. A thick layer is not more effective than a thin layer.

DO NOT bandage the area unless directed by your doctor.

 If your medication is a lotion or a suspension SHAKE the container well before applying.

 If your medication is an aerosol spray, SHAKE the container well before applying and hold the container straight up, about 6-8 inches from the affected skin area and spray for 2-3 seconds.

DO NOT apply any other creams, lotions or cosmetics on top of or beneath the medication.

 Call your doctor if the condition persists or becomes worse, or if you have a constant irritation, such as burning or itching that was not present before you started this medication.

DO NOT keep or use outdated medication. Keep all medication out of the reach of children.

In case of accidental ingestion, call your doctor or poison control center immediately.

HOW TO USE RECTAL PREPARATIONS

HOW TO USE RECTAL CREAMS:

 Wash your hands with soap and water before and after using this medication.

Wash and pat dry the rectal area before using this medication.

Application to the outer rectal area:

– Remove the cap from the tube and apply the medicine to the rectal area. Rub in gently.

You may use toilet paper or a finger cot to avoid putting the medication directly on your finger.

Application into the anorectal area:

– Remove the cap from the tube and attach the plastic applicator tip.

– Squeeze out a small amount of medicine and spread it around to lubricate the applicator tip.

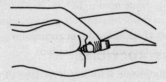

– Lie down on your side and insert the applicator tip gently into the rectum. Gently squeeze the tube to administer the medicine.

Remain on your side for a few minutes before getting up.

After using this medication, remove the applicator tip from the tube and wash it with soap and water.

Place the cap on the tube and close tightly.

HOW TO USE RECTAL SUPPOSITORIES:

Wash your hands with soap and water before and after using this medication.

Wash and pat dry the rectal area before using this medication.

Remove the wrapper and moisten the suppository with lukewarm water to soften it if needed.

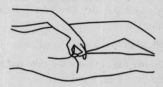

Lie down on your side.

Use your finger to push the pointed end of the suppository just inside the rectum. You may use toilet paper or a finger cot to avoid direct finger contact.

If the suppository is too soft to insert, cool it in the refrigerator or run under cold water before removing the wrapper.

Suppositories need to be stored in a cool place to avoid melting. Some need to be kept in a refrigerator. If you can not determine the correct storage requirements for this product check with your pharmacist.

SPECIAL INSTRUCTIONS:

This medication is for RECTAL USE ONLY.

Call your doctor if the condition persists or becomes worse, or if you have a constant irritation, such as burning or itching that was not present before you started this medication.

DO NOT keep or use outdated medication. Keep all medication out of the reach of children.

In case of accidental ingestion, call your doctor or poison control center immediately.

AMPICILLIN
Ampicillin, Omnipen, Polycillin, Principen, Totacillin

THIS MEDICATION IS USED:

To treat infections.

PROPER USE OF THIS MEDICATION:

 Unless your doctor has told you differently, this medicine should be taken on an empty stomach with a glass of water at least 1 hour before or 2 hours after a meal.

 If you are taking the liquid form, it should be stored in the refrigerator and used within 14 days. The contents should be shaken well just before measuring the dose. There are special measuring devices available, ask your pharmacist if you want one.

SPECIAL INSTRUCTIONS:

 The recommended length of treatment is 7-10 days. You should take all the medication unless otherwise instructed by your doctor.

 If you experience diarrhea while taking this medicine, DO NOT take any antidiarrheal medicine without first asking your doctor or pharmacist.

If you miss a dose, take the missed dose as soon as possible. But if it is almost time for your next dose (within 2 hours), DOUBLE that dose. Then go back to your regular dosing schedule.

DO NOT keep or use outdated medication. Keep all medication out of the reach of children.

POSSIBLE SIDE EFFECTS:

 Be sure to tell your doctor if the following occur: skin rash, hives or itching, shortness of breath or wheezing, swelling of the face, prolonged nausea, vomiting or diarrhea, black tongue, or persistent sore throat or fever.

AMOXICILLIN
Amoxil, Polymox, Trimox, Wymox

THIS MEDICATION IS USED:

To treat infections.

PROPER USE OF THIS MEDICATION:

 This medication should be taken with a glass of water and it can be taken with or without food.

 If you are taking the liquid form, it should be stored in the refrigerator and used within 14 days. The contents should be shaken well just before measuring the dose. There are special measuring devices available, ask your pharmacist for one.

 If you are taking the chewable form, it should be chewed well before swallowing.

SPECIAL INSTRUCTIONS:

 The recommended length of treatment is 7-10 days. You should take all the medication unless otherwise instructed by your doctor.

 If you experience diarrhea while taking this medicine, DO NOT take any antidiarrheal medicine without first asking your doctor or pharmacist.

If you miss a dose, take the missed dose as soon as possible. But if it is almost time for your next dose (within 2 hours), DOUBLE that dose. Then go back to your regular dosing schedule.

DO NOT keep or use outdated medication. Keep all medication out of the reach of children.

POSSIBLE SIDE EFFECTS:

 Be sure to tell your doctor if the following occur: skin rash, hives or itching, shortness of breath or wheezing, swelling of the face, prolonged nausea, vomiting or diarrhea, black tongue, or persistent sore throat or fever.

PENICILLIN G, PENTIDS

THIS MEDICATION IS USED:

To treat infections.

PROPER USE OF THIS MEDICINE:

 Unless your doctor has told you differently, this medicine should be taken on an empty stomach with a glass of water at least 1 hour before or 2 hours after a meal.

DO NOT take this medication with any acidic fruit drinks (i.e. orange juice).

 If you are taking the liquid form, it should be stored in the refrigerator and used within 14 days. The contents should be shaken well just before measuring the dose. There are special measuring devices available, ask your pharmacist if you want one.

SPECIAL INSTRUCTIONS:

 The recommended length of treatment is 7-10 days. You should take all the medication unless otherwise instructed by your doctor.

 If you experience diarrhea while taking this medicine, DO NOT take any antidiarrheal medicine without first asking your doctor or pharmacist.

If you miss a dose, take the missed dose as soon as possible. But if it is almost time for your next dose (within 2 hours), DOUBLE that dose. Then go back to your regular dosing schedule.

DO NOT keep or use outdated medication. Keep all medication out of the reach of children.

POSSIBLE SIDE EFFECTS:

 Be sure to tell your doctor if the following occur: skin rash, hives or itching, shortness of breath or wheezing, swelling of the face, prolonged nausea, vomiting or diarrhea, black tongue, or persistent sore throat or fever.

PENICILLIN DERIVATIVES

Beepen-VK, Betapen-VK, Cloxacillin, Dicloxacillin, Dynapen,
Ledercillin-VK, Pathocil, Pen-Vee K, Penicillin VK, Tegopen,
V-Cillin K, Veetids

THIS MEDICATION IS USED:

To treat infections.

PROPER USE OF THIS MEDICATION:

 Some forms of this medication should be taken on an empty stomach with a glass of water, others may be taken without regard to food. If you have not been told which is best, check with your doctor or pharmacist.

 If this medication upsets your stomach, it may be taken with food.

 If you are taking the liquid form, it should be stored in the refrigerator and used within 14 days. The contents should be shaken well just before measuring the dose. There are special measuring devices available, ask your pharmacist if you want one.

SPECIAL INSTRUCTIONS:

 The recommended length of treatment is 7-10 days. You should take all the medication unless otherwise instructed by your doctor.

 If you experience diarrhea while taking this medicine, DO NOT take any antidiarrheal medicine without first asking your doctor or pharmacist.

If you miss a dose, take the missed dose as soon as possible. But if it is almost time for your next dose (within 2 hours), DOUBLE that dose. Then go back to your regular dosing schedule.

DO NOT keep or use outdated medicine. Keep this medicine at room temperature, in its original container and out of the reach of children.

If the medicine is in liquid form, keep it in the refrigerator and discard it after 14 days.

POSSIBLE SIDE EFFECTS:

 Be sure to tell your doctor if the following occur: skin rash, hives or itching, shortness of breath or wheezing, swelling of the face, prolonged nausea, vomiting or diarrhea, black tongue, or persistent sore throat or fever.

ERYTHROMYCIN

E-Mycin, E-Mycin E, E.E.S., E.E.S. Filmtab, Ery-Tab Enteric Coated, Eryc, Eryped, Erythrocin Stearate, Erythromycin, Erythromycin Estolate, Erythromycin Ethylsuccinate, Erythromycin Stearate, Ilosone, PCE, Wyamycin S

THIS MEDICATION IS USED:

To treat infections.

PROPER USE OF THIS MEDICATION:

 Some forms of this medication should be taken on an empty stomach with a glass of water, others may be taken without regards to food. If you have not been told which is best, check with your doctor or pharmacist.

 If you are taking the liquid form, some may be stored in the refrigerator, others may be kept at room temperature. If you are not sure as to how to store your medicine, ask your pharmacist. The contents should be shaken well just before measuring the dose. There are special measuring devices available, ask your pharmacist for one.

If you are taking the chewable form, it should be chewed well before swallowing.

The pellet, film and enteric coated forms should be swallowed whole, NOT crushed or chewed.

SPECIAL INSTRUCTIONS:

 The recommended length of treatment is 7-10 days. You should take all the medication unless otherwise instructed by your doctor.

If you experience diarrhea while taking this medicine, DO NOT take any antidiarrheal medicine without first asking your doctor or pharmacist.

You should talk with your doctor before taking the following prescription medications: astemizole (Hismanal) and terfenadine (Seldane, Seldane-D).

If you miss a dose, take the missed dose as soon as possible. But if it is almost time for your next dose (within 2 hours), DOUBLE that dose. Then go back to your regular dosing schedule.

DO NOT keep or use outdated medication. Keep all medication out of the reach of children.

POSSIBLE SIDE EFFECTS:

 Be sure to tell your doctor if the following occur: prolonged or severe nausea, vomiting or diarrhea.

SULFONAMIDE
Bactrim, Cotrim SMZ-TMP, Gantanol, Gantrisin, Septra, Sulfamethoxazole, Sulfamethoxazole-Trimethoprim, Sulfisoxazole

THIS MEDICATION IS USED:

To treat infections.

PROPER USE OF THIS MEDICATION:

 Take this medicine with a glass of water. If it upsets your stomach you may take it with food.

 The liquid form of this medication should be shaken well just before measuring the dose. There are special measuring devices available, ask your pharmacist if you want one.

SPECIAL INSTRUCTIONS:

 The recommended length of treatment is 7-10 days. You should take all the medication unless otherwise instructed by your doctor.

It is recommended that you drink lots of fluids while you are taking this medication.

 This medicine may make your skin more sensitive to sunlight or sunlamps. Ask your pharmacist about a suitable sunblock product (of at least SPF 15) to minimize problems during exposure.

 If you experience diarrhea while taking this medicine, DO NOT take any antidiarrheal medicine without first asking your doctor or pharmacist.

If you miss a dose, take the missed dose as soon as possible. But if it is almost time for your next dose (within 2 hours), DOUBLE that dose. Then go back to your regular dosing schedule.

DO NOT keep or use outdated medication. Keep all medication out of the reach of children.

POSSIBLE SIDE EFFECTS:

 Be sure to tell your doctor if the following occur: skin rash, hives or itching, prolonged nausea, vomiting or diarrhea, sore throat, fever, unusual bleeding or bruising, or yellow coloration of the eyes or skin.

TETRACYCLINE
Achromycin V, Declomycin, Oxytetracycline, Panmycin, Sumycin, Terramycin

THIS MEDICATION IS USED:

To treat infections.

PROPER USE OF THIS MEDICATION:

 Unless your doctor has told you differently, this medicine should be taken on an empty stomach with a glass of water at least 1 hour before or 2 hours after a meal. If it upsets your stomach, you may take it with food.

 DO NOT take this medication at the same time as milk or other dairy products.

 If you are taking the liquid form, the contents should be shaken well just before measuring the dose. There are special measuring devices available, ask your pharmacist if you want one.

 DO NOT take antacids or iron supplements within 2 hours of taking this medication.

SPECIAL INSTRUCTIONS:

 The recommended length of treatment is 7-10 days. You should take all the medication unless otherwise instructed by your doctor.

 This medication may make your skin more sensitive to sunlight or sunlamps. Ask your pharmacist about a suitable sunblock product (of at least SPF 15) to reduce exposure problems.

If you miss a dose, take the missed dose as soon as possible. But if it is almost time for your next dose (within 2 hours), DOUBLE that dose. Then go back to your regular dosing schedule.

DO NOT keep or use outdated medication. Keep all medication out of the reach of children.

POSSIBLE SIDE EFFECTS:

Be sure to tell your doctor if the following occur: cramps, nausea or vomiting, rectal itch or sores on the tongue or mouth.

CEPHALOSPORIN

Anspor, Biocef, Ceclor, Ceftin, Cefzil, Cephadrine, Cephalexin, Duricef, Keflet, Keflex, Keftab, Ultracef, Velosef

THIS MEDICATION IS USED:

To treat infections.

PROPER USE OF THIS MEDICATION:

 Take this medicine with a glass of water. If it upsets your stomach you may take it with food.

 If you are taking the liquid form, it should be stored in the refrigerator and used within 14 days. The contents should be shaken well just before measuring the dose. There are special measuring devices available, ask your pharmacist if you want one.

SPECIAL INSTRUCTIONS:

 The recommended length of treatment is 7-10 days. You should take all the medication unless otherwise instructed by your doctor.

 If you experience diarrhea while taking this medicine, DO NOT take any antidiarrheal medicine without first asking your doctor or pharmacist.

If you miss a dose, take the missed dose as soon as possible. But if it is almost time for your next dose (within 2 hours), DOUBLE that dose. Then go back to your regular dosing schedule.

DO NOT keep or use outdated medication. Keep all medication out of the reach of children.

POSSIBLE SIDE EFFECTS:

 Be sure to tell your doctor if the following occur: skin rash, hives or itching, shortness of breath or wheezing, swelling of the face, prolonged nausea, vomiting or diarrhea, black tongue, or persistent sore throat or fever.

DOXYCYCLINE
Doryx, Doxycycline, Monodox, Vibra-Tabs, Vibramycin

THIS MEDICATION IS USED:

To treat infections.

PROPER USE OF THIS MEDICATION:

 Unless your doctor has told you differently, this medicine should be taken on an empty stomach with a glass of water. You may take it with food if it upsets your stomach.

 If you are taking the liquid form, it should be stored at room temperature. The contents should be shaken well just before measuring the dose. There are special measuring devices available, ask your pharmacist if you want one.

 The contents of the pellet form should NOT be crushed or chewed.

DO NOT take antacids or iron supplements within 2 hours of taking this medication.

SPECIAL INSTRUCTIONS:

 The recommended length of treatment is 7-10 days. You should take all the medication unless otherwise instructed by your doctor.

 This medication may make your skin more sensitive to sunlight or sunlamps. Ask your pharmacist about a suitable sunblock product (of at least SPF 15) to reduce exposure problems.

If you miss a dose, take the missed dose as soon as possible. But if it is almost time for your next dose (within 2 hours), and your dosing schedule is:

Once daily – space the missed dose and the next dose 10-12 hours apart

Twice daily – space the missed dose and the next dose 5-6 hours apart.

Then go back to your regular dosing schedule.

DO NOT keep or use outdated medication. Keep all medication out of the reach of children.

POSSIBLE SIDE EFFECTS:

 Be sure to tell your doctor if the following occur: cramps, nausea or vomiting, rectal itch or sores on the tongue or mouth.

ANTIHISTAMINE

Benadryl, Clemastine, Cyproheptadine, Diphenhydramine, Optimine, Periactin, Phenergan Fortis, Phenergan Liquid, Polaramine, Promethazine Liquid, Tavist, Temaril, Temaril Spansule

THIS MEDICATION IS USED:

To relieve the runny nose, watery eyes and sneezing of colds and hay fever. Some forms may also be used for allergic reactions.

PROPER USE OF THIS MEDICATION:

 Take this medicine with a glass of water, if it upsets your stomach you may take it with food.

If you are taking the liquid form, you may measure the dose by using a special measuring device. Ask your pharmacist if you want one.

 The controlled release forms should be swallowed whole, NOT crushed or chewed.

SPECIAL INSTRUCTIONS:

 You may experience dizziness, blurred vision or drowsiness from this medicine. If you do, be careful driving or performing hazardous tasks.

 Alcoholic beverages can increase the drowsiness.

If your mouth becomes dry, you may suck on hard candy, chew gum or use a saliva substitute.

 This medicine may make your skin more sensitive to sunlight or sunlamps. Ask your pharmacist about a suitable sunblock product (of at least SPF 15) to minimize problems during exposure.

 You should NOT take nonprescription cough/cold products without asking your doctor or pharmacist.

If you miss a dose of this medicine, take it as soon as possible. But, if it is almost time for your next dose, skip the missed dose and go back to your regular dose. DO NOT take a double dose.

DO NOT keep or use outdated medication. Keep all medication out of the reach of children.

POSSIBLE SIDE EFFECTS:

 Be sure to tell your doctor if the following occur: drowsiness, blurred vision, dry mouth, headache, mental confusion, loss of appetite.

CORTICOSTEROID (ORAL INHALER)

Aerobid Inhaler, Aerobid-M Inhaler, Azmacort Inhaler, Beclovent Inhaler, Decadron Respihaler, Vanceril Inhaler

THIS MEDICATION IS USED:

To prevent asthma attacks.

PROPER USE OF THIS MEDICATION:

BE SURE the canister is properly inserted into the inhaler unit.

 REMOVE dust cap and SHAKE the unit WELL.

Hold the inhaler with the nozzle down, unless your doctor has told you otherwise.

Unless your doctor has told you otherwise, exhale fully and place mouthpiece into your mouth with your lips closed around it and your tongue flat.

As you take a deep breath, squeeze the can and mouthpiece together at exactly the same time.

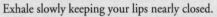

Continue taking a deep breath and hold it for as long as comfortable.

Exhale slowly keeping your lips nearly closed.

 If your doctor has instructed you to use more than one inhalation at each use, wait a minute between inhalations, repeat the above steps. Be sure to shake the unit before each inhalation.

After the prescribed amount of inhalations, rinse out your mouth with water.

SPECIAL INSTRUCTIONS:

Notify your doctor if your mouth becomes sore or develops a rash.

KEEP THE MOUTHPIECE CLEAN. At least once daily, wash the mouthpiece with soap and hot water. Rinse thoroughly and allow to dry.

The contents of the can are under pressure. DO NOT puncture or throw it into an incinerator.

When not using the inhaler, store it with the dust cap on the mouthpiece. This will prevent dirt and dust from getting into the mouthpiece.

Instructions for each brand of inhaler are similar, but slightly different. Read them carefully and follow the directions. If you have any questions, ask your doctor or pharmacist.

Proper control of your condition requires you to use this medicine as instructed at the same time every day, DO NOT skip a dose nor stop using the medicine without asking your doctor.

It is important that you continue using this medicine as your doctor has instructed. It may take several days before improvement is noticed.

If you are also using a bronchodilator inhaler, be sure to use it first. Wait 2-3 minutes then use this medication.

If you miss a dose of this medicine, use it as soon as possible. But, if it is almost time for your next dose, skip the missed dose and go back to your regular dose. DO NOT take a double dose.

DO NOT keep or use outdated medicine. Keep this medicine at room temperature, in its original container and out of the reach of children.

POSSIBLE SIDE EFFECTS:

Be sure to tell your doctor if the following occur: diarrhea, nausea or vomiting, persistent sore throat, muscle cramps or pain, headache, dizziness, nervousness or blurred vision.

BRONCHODILATOR, BETA-ADRENERGIC (ORAL)

Albuterol, Alupent, Brethine, Bricanyl, Metaprel,
Metaproterenol, Proventil, Proventil Repetabs, Ventolin

THIS MEDICATION IS USED:

To treat the symptoms of bronchial asthma, chronic bronchitis and emphysema.

PROPER USE OF THIS MEDICATION:

 Take this medicine with a glass of water. If it upsets your stomach you may take it with food.

 The controlled release forms should be swallowed whole, NOT crushed or chewed.

If you are taking the liquid form, there are special measuring devices available to measure your dose, ask your pharmacist if you want one.

SPECIAL INSTRUCTIONS:

 Proper control of your condition requires you to take this medicine as instructed at the same time every day, DO NOT skip a dose nor stop taking the medicine without asking your doctor.

 DO NOT take nonprescription cough/cold, hayfever or sleep aid products without asking your doctor or pharmacist.

 Cigarette smoking will affect your condition. DO NOT increase the amount of cigarettes you smoke. Instead, try to quit smoking, your doctor or pharmacist can explain various methods.

If you miss a dose of this medicine, take it as soon as possible. But, if it is almost time for your next dose, skip the missed dose and go back to your regular dose. DO NOT take a double dose.

DO NOT keep or use outdated medication. Keep all medication out of the reach of children.

POSSIBLE SIDE EFFECTS:

 Be sure to tell your doctor if the following occur: chest pain, severe dizziness or headache, irregular or pounding heartbeat.

BRONCHODILATOR, XANTHINE

Bronkodyl, Choledyl, Choledyl SA, Dyflex, Dyphylline, Elixophyllin, Lufyllin, Marax, Marax DF, Quibron-T, Quibron-T SR, Respbid, Slo-Bid, Slo-Phyllin, T-Phyl, Theo-24, Theo-Dur, Theochron, Theoclear, Theolair, Theolair-SR, Theophylline, Theostat, Uniphyl

THIS MEDICATION IS USED:

To treat the symptoms of bronchial asthma, chronic bronchitis and emphysema.

PROPER USE OF THIS MEDICATION:

Some forms of this medication work best when taken on an empty stomach with a glass of water. Others may be taken without regards to food. If you have not been told which is best, check with your doctor or pharmacist.

If this medication upsets your stomach you may take it with food unless otherwise instructed.

The controlled release forms should be swallowed whole, NOT crushed or chewed.

Some of the liquid forms require the contents to be shaken well just before measuring the dose. There are special measuring devices available, ask your pharmacist if you want one.

SPECIAL INSTRUCTIONS:

Proper control of your condition requires you to take this medicine as instructed at the same time every day, DO NOT skip a dose nor stop taking the medicine without asking your doctor.

DO NOT take nonprescription cough/cold, hay fever or sleep aid products without asking your doctor or pharmacist.

It is recommended that you drink lots of fluids while taking this medication.

Avoid drinking large amounts of caffeine containing beverages (i.e. cocoa, coffee, cola or tea) while taking this medication, since an increase in nervousness is possible.

Cigarette smoking will affect your condition as well as your medication. DO NOT increase the amount of cigarettes you smoke. Instead, try to quit smoking, your doctor or pharmacist can explain various methods.

If you miss a dose of this medicine, take it as soon as possible. But, if it is almost time for your next dose, skip the missed dose and go back to your regular dose. DO NOT take a double dose.

DO NOT keep or use outdated medication. Keep all medication out of the reach of children.

POSSIBLE SIDE EFFECTS:

Be sure to tell your doctor if the following occur: unusual heartbeat, thirst, urination, tiredness or weakness, mental confusion or flu-like symptoms.

ACETAMINOPHEN – NARCOTIC

Acetaminophen w/Codeine, Acetaminophen w/Hydrocodone, Anexsia, Bancap-HC, Darvocet-N, Lorcet, Lorcet Plus, Lortab, Oxycodone w/Acetaminophen, Percocet, Phenaphen 650 w/Codeine, Phenaphen w/Codeine, Propacet, Propoxyphene Napsylate w/Apap, Roxicet, Talacen, Tylenol w/Codeine, Tylox, Vicodin, Vicodines, Zydone

THIS MEDICATION IS USED:

To relieve pain.

PROPER USE OF THIS MEDICATION:

 Take this medicine with a glass of water. If it upsets your stomach you may take it with food.

 Some of the liquid forms require the contents to be shaken well just before measuring the dose. There are special measuring devices available, ask your pharmacist if you want one.

SPECIAL INSTRUCTIONS:

 You may experience dizziness, blurred vision or drowsiness from this medicine. If you do, be careful driving or performing hazardous tasks.

Alcoholic beverages can increase the drowsiness.

 If taken for a few days, you may experience some constipation. You should increase the amount of bulk in your diet (bran, psyllium or fresh fruits) and drink lots of fluids.

 DO NOT take nonprescription ibuprofen, aspirin or acetaminophen products while taking this drug without checking with your doctor or pharmacist.

If you miss a dose of this medicine, take it as soon as possible. But, if it is almost time for your next dose, skip the missed dose and go back to your regular dose. DO NOT take a double dose.

DO NOT keep or use outdated medication. Keep all medication out of the reach of children.

POSSIBLE SIDE EFFECTS:

 Be sure to tell your doctor if the following occur: drowsiness, dizziness or lightheadedness, nausea or vomiting, heartburn or indigestion, difficult breathing, unusual heartbeat, sweating, excitement, skin rash, yellow coloration of eyes or skin or blue coloration of the fingernails.

ASPIRIN – NARCOTIC

Aspirin w/Codeine, Empirin W/Codeine, Oxycodone w/Aspirin,
Percodan, Percodan-Demi, Synalgos/DC

THIS MEDICATION IS USED:

To relieve pain.

PROPER USE OF THIS MEDICATION:

 Take this medication with food and a glass of water to avoid upsetting your stomach.

SPECIAL INSTRUCTIONS:

 You may experience dizziness, blurred vision or drowsiness from this medicine. If you do, be careful driving or performing hazardous tasks.

Alcoholic beverages can increase drowsiness.

 DO NOT take nonprescription ibuprofen, aspirin or acetaminophen products while taking this drug without checking with your doctor or pharmacist.

 If taken for a few days, you may experience some constipation. You should increase the amount of bulk in your diet (bran, psyllium and fresh fruits) and drink lots of fluids.

 Discard doses that have a strong vinegar odor. The aspirin has decomposed.

If you miss a dose of this medicine, take it as soon as possible. But, if it is almost time for your next dose, skip the missed dose and go back to your regular dose. DO NOT take a double dose.

DO NOT keep or use outdated medication. Keep all medication out of the reach of children.

POSSIBLE SIDE EFFECTS:

 Be sure to tell your doctor if the following occur: drowsiness, dizziness or lightheadedness, nausea or vomiting, heartburn or stomach cramps, difficult breathing, unusual heartbeat, sweating, excitement, skin rash, ringing or buzzing in the ears, black, tarry or bloody stools.

NARCOTIC

Codeine, Darvon, Darvon-N, Demerol, Dilaudid, Hydrocodone, Meperidine MS, Morphine, Contin, Oramorph SR, Propoxyphene HCL, Propoxyphene Napsylate, Roxanol, Roxanol SR, Talwin NX

THIS MEDICATION IS USED:

For the relief of pain.

PROPER USE OF THIS MEDICATION:

 Take this medicine with a glass of water. If it upsets your stomach you may take it with food.

 Some of the liquid forms require the contents to be shaken well just before measuring the dose. There are special measuring devices available, ask your pharmacist if you want one.

 The controlled release forms should be swallowed whole, NOT crushed or chewed.

SPECIAL INSTRUCTIONS:

 You may experience dizziness, blurred vision or drowsiness from this medicine. If you do, be careful driving or performing hazardous tasks.

Alcoholic beverages can increase the drowsiness.

 If taken for a few days, you may experience some constipation. You should increase the amount of bulk in your diet (bran, psyllium, and fresh fruits) and drink lots of fluids.

 DO NOT take nonprescription ibuprofen, aspirin or acetaminophen products while taking this drug without checking with your doctor or pharmacist.

If you miss a dose of this medicine, take it as soon as possible. But, if it is almost time for your next dose, skip the missed dose and go back to your regular dosing schedule. DO NOT take a double dose.

DO NOT keep or use outdated medication. Keep all medication out of the reach of children.

POSSIBLE SIDE EFFECTS:

 Be sure to tell your doctor if the following occur: drowsiness, dizziness or lightheadedness, nausea or vomiting, heartburn or indigestion, difficult breathing, unusual heartbeat, sweating, excitement or skin rash.

ANTI-INFLAMMATORY, NONSTEROIDAL

Advil Children's, Anaprox, Ansaid, Feldene, Fenoprofen, Ibuprofen, Lodine, Meclofenamate, Meclomen, Motrin, Nalfon, Naprosyn, Orudis, Pediaprofen, Piroxicam, Ponstel, Relafen, Rufen, Tolectin, Tolmetin

THIS MEDICATION IS USED:

For the relief of pain. It can also be used to reduce fever, to treat menstrual pain and to relieve swelling in certain kinds of arthritis.

PROPER USE OF THIS MEDICATION:

Some types of this medicine can be taken with food or an antacid followed by a glass of water to reduce the chance of stomach upset. If you have not been told which is best, check with your doctor or pharmacist.

If you are taking the liquid form, the contents should be shaken well just before measuring the dose. There are special measuring devices available, ask your pharmacist if you want one.

SPECIAL INSTRUCTIONS:

If this medicine is used for arthritis, it must be taken regularly as ordered by your doctor.

DO NOT take nonprescription ibuprofen, aspirin or acetaminophen products while taking this drug without checking with your doctor or pharmacist.

You may experience dizziness, blurred vision or drowsiness from this medicine. If you do, be careful driving or performing hazardous tasks.

If you miss a dose of this medicine, take it as soon as possible. But, if it is almost time for your next dose, skip the missed dose and take your regular dose. DO NOT take a double dose.

DO NOT keep or use outdated medication. Keep all medication out of the reach of children.

POSSIBLE SIDE EFFECTS:

 Be sure to tell your doctor if any of the following occur: skin rash, ringing or buzzing in the ears, changed vision, stomach pain or nausea, persistent sore throat or fever, black, tarry or bloody stools, unusual weight gain or edema in the extremities or difficulty in breathing.

VOLTAREN

THIS MEDICATION IS USED:

For the relief of pain and swelling in certain kinds of arthritis.

PROPER USE OF THIS MEDICATION:

This medication should be taken with a glass of water.

This medication is enteric coated. It should be swallowed whole, NOT crushed or chewed.

SPECIAL INSTRUCTIONS:

This medicine is used for arthritis, it must be taken regularly as ordered by your doctor.

DO NOT take nonprescription ibuprofen, aspirin or acetaminophen products while taking this drug without checking with your doctor or pharmacist.

You may experience dizziness, blurred vision or drowsiness from this medicine. If you do, be careful driving or performing hazardous tasks.

If you miss a dose of this medicine, take it as soon as possible. But, if it is almost time for your next dose, skip the missed dose and take your regular dose. DO NOT take a double dose.

DO NOT keep or use outdated medication. Keep all medication out of the reach of children.

POSSIBLE SIDE EFFECTS:

Be sure to tell your doctor if any of the following occur: skin rash, ringing or buzzing in the ears, changed vision, stomach pain or nausea, persistent sore throat or fever, black, tarry or bloody stools, unusual weight gain or edema in the extremities or difficulty in breathing.

SULINDAC, CLINORIL

THIS MEDICATION IS USED:

For the relief of pain and swelling in certain kinds of arthritis and other conditions such as bursitis and tendinitis.

PROPER USE OF THIS MEDICATION:

 This medication should be taken with food followed by a glass of water to reduce the chance of stomach upset.

SPECIAL INSTRUCTIONS:

If this medicine is used for arthritis, it must be taken regularly as ordered by your doctor.

 DO NOT take nonprescription ibuprofen, aspirin or acetaminophen products while taking this drug without checking with your doctor or pharmacist.

 You may experience dizziness, blurred vision or drowsiness from this medicine. If you do, be careful driving or performing hazardous tasks.

If you miss a dose of this medicine, take it as soon as possible. But, if it is almost time for your next dose, skip the missed dose and take your regular dose. DO NOT take a double dose.

DO NOT keep or use outdated medication. Keep all medication out of the reach of children.

POSSIBLE SIDE EFFECTS:

 Be sure to tell your doctor if any of the following occur: skin rash, ringing or buzzing in the ears, changed vision, stomach pain or nausea, persistent sore throat or fever, black, tarry or bloody stools, unusual weight gain or edema in the extremities or difficulty in breathing.

INDOMETHACIN
Indocin, Indocin SR

THIS MEDICATION IS USED:

For the relief of pain and swelling in certain kinds of arthritis and other conditions such as bursitis and tendinitis.

PROPER USE OF THIS MEDICATION:

 This medication should be taken with food or an antacid followed by a glass of water to reduce the chance of stomach upset.

 If you are taking the liquid form, the contents should be shaken well just before measuring the dose. There are special measuring devices available, ask your pharmacist if you want one.

 The controlled release pellet form should be swallowed whole, NOT crushed or chewed or dissolved in liquid.

SPECIAL INSTRUCTIONS:

If this medicine is used for arthritis, it must be taken regularly as ordered by your doctor.

 DO NOT take nonprescription ibuprofen, aspirin or acetaminophen products while taking this drug without checking with your doctor or pharmacist.

 You may experience dizziness, blurred vision or drowsiness from this medicine. If you do, be careful driving or performing hazardous tasks.

If you miss a dose of this medicine, take it as soon as possible. But, if it is almost time for your next dose, skip the missed dose and take your regular dose. DO NOT take a double dose.

DO NOT keep or use outdated medication. Keep all medication out of the reach of children.

POSSIBLE SIDE EFFECTS:

 Be sure to tell your doctor if any of the following occur: skin rash, ringing or buzzing in the ears, changed vision, stomach pain or nausea, persistent sore throat or fever, black, tarry or bloody stools, unusual weight gain or edema in the extremities or difficulty in breathing.

CORTICOSTEROID

Aristocort, Celestone, Cortef, Cortisone, Decadron, Deltasone, Dexamethasone, Hexadrol, Hydrocortisone, Kenacort, Medrol, Methylprednisolone, Meticorten, Orasone, Prednisolone, Prednisone, Prelone, Triamcinolone

THIS MEDICATION IS USED:

To help relieve the symptoms of severe allergies, skin conditions, and pain due to certain types of arthritis or inflammation.

PROPER USE OF THIS MEDICATION:

 Take this medicine with a glass of water. If it upsets your stomach you may take it with food.

 Some of the liquid forms require the contents to be shaken well just before measuring the dose. There are special measuring devices available, ask your pharmacist if you want one.

SPECIAL INSTRUCTIONS:

 If you continue to have stomach upset while taking this medication, you should tell your doctor.

 Proper control of your condition requires you to take this medicine as instructed at the same time every day, DO NOT skip a dose nor stop taking the medicine without asking your doctor.

 You should NOT take aspirin products or drink alcohol while taking this medicine without asking your doctor, since stomach upset might occur.

If you miss a dose of this medication and your dosing schedule is:

– One dose every other day: Take the missed dose as soon as possible, ONLY if you remember the same morning. If you remember later in the day, take it the next morning and then skip a day.

– Once a day dose: Take the missed dose as soon as possible. But, if it is almost time for your next dose, skip the

missed dose and go back to your regular dose. DO NOT take a double dose.

- Several doses a day: Take the missed dose as soon as possible. If it is time for your next dose double that dose.

DO NOT keep or use outdated medication. Keep all medication out of the reach of children.

POSSIBLE SIDE EFFECTS:

 Be sure to tell your doctor if the following occur: muscle cramps or pains, swelling of the face, hands or feet, nausea, vomiting, black or tarry stools and mood or skin changes.

SULFONYLUREA

Chlorpropamide, Diabeta, Diabinese, Dymelor, Glynase, Micronase, Oramide, Orinase, Tolamide, Tolazamide, Tolbutamide, Tolinase

THIS MEDICATION IS USED:

To treat diabetes.

PROPER USE OF THIS MEDICATION:

 This medication should be taken with a glass of water and it can be taken with or without food.

The morning dose should be taken with breakfast.

SPECIAL INSTRUCTIONS:

 Proper control of your condition requires you to take this medicine as instructed at the same time every day, DO NOT skip a dose nor stop taking the medicine without asking your doctor.

Since this medicine does not cure but helps to control your condition, you should continue to take it even if you are feeling well.

 DO NOT take nonprescription cough/cold, aspirin or diet products without asking your doctor or pharmacist.

 DO NOT drink alcoholic beverages before checking with your doctor.

 Call your doctor if you develop any signs of hyperglycemia (high blood sugar) such as: excessive thirst or urination, high glucose or ketones in the urine or blood, fast breathing or dry skin.

Call your doctor if you develop any signs of hypoglycemia (low blood sugar) such as: nervousness, sweating and increased hunger or heart rate.

 Your pharmacist can advise you on the various types of diabetic testing products on the market and their proper procedures for use.

If you miss a dose of this medicine, take it as soon as possible. But, if it is almost time for your next dose, skip the missed dose and go back to your regular dose. DO NOT take a double dose.

DO NOT keep or use outdated medication. Keep all medication out of the reach of children.

POSSIBLE SIDE EFFECTS:

 Be sure to tell your doctor if the following occur: yellow coloring of the skin or eyes, unusual bruising or bleeding or recurrent sore throat or fever.

GLUCOTROL

THIS MEDICATION IS USED:

To treat diabetes.

PROPER USE OF THIS MEDICATION:

 This medication should be taken with a glass of water 30 minutes before meals.

SPECIAL INSTRUCTIONS:

 Proper control of your condition requires you to take this medicine as instructed at the same time every day, DO NOT skip a dose nor stop taking the medicine without asking your doctor.

Since this medicine does not cure but helps to control your condition, you should continue to take it even if you are feeling well.

 DO NOT take nonprescription cough/cold, aspirin or diet products without asking your doctor or pharmacist.

DO NOT drink alcoholic beverages before checking with your doctor.

 Call your doctor if you develop any signs of hyperglycemia (high blood sugar) such as: excessive thirst or urination, high glucose or ketones in the urine or blood, fast breathing or dry skin.

Call your doctor if you develop any signs of hypoglycemia (low blood sugar) such as: nervousness, sweating and increased hunger or heart rate.

 Your pharmacist can advise you on the various types of diabetic testing products on the market and their proper procedures for use.

If you miss a dose of this medicine, take it as soon as possible. But, if it is almost time for your next dose, skip the

missed dose and go back to your regular dose. DO NOT take a double dose.

DO NOT keep or use outdated medication. Keep all medication out of the reach of children.

POSSIBLE SIDE EFFECTS:

 Be sure to tell your doctor if the following occur: yellow coloring of the skin or eyes, unusual bruising or bleeding or recurrent sore throat or fever.

NITROGLYCERIN SUBLINGUAL
Isonate Sublingual, Isordil Sublingual, Isosorbide Sublingual, Nitrostat Sublingual, Sorbitrate Sublingual

THIS MEDICATION IS USED:

To relieve angina attacks.

PROPER USE OF THIS MEDICATION:

 At the first sign of an attack, sit down as soon as possible.

 Place the tablet under your tongue or in the pouch of your cheek until it is dissolved. Wait a few minutes before swallowing or drinking.

This medication should be effective within 3 doses or 15 minutes. If the first tablet does not relieve the pain in 5 minutes, a second tablet may be used. This can again be repeated in another 5 minutes. If the chest pain is not relieved after 3 doses or 15 minutes, your doctor or ambulance service should be contacted.

SPECIAL INSTRUCTIONS:

 It is important that you take this medicine exactly as your doctor has instructed.

DO NOT eat or drink while the tablet is dissolving in your mouth.

 DO NOT swallow, chew or crush this tablet.

To prevent loss of potency, keep the tablets in original container. Close tightly after each use.

When opened for the first time make a note on the bottle of the date. If all tablets are not used within 6 months consider obtaining more.

 Store this medicine in a cool dry place, but NOT in the refrigerator or medicine cabinet.

 Headache, flushing of the face or dizziness may occur with the first few doses. This is normal and should stop. If these effects continue, tell your doctor.

DO NOT keep or use outdated medication. Keep all medication out of the reach of children.

POSSIBLE SIDE EFFECTS:

 Be sure to tell your doctor if the following occur: persistent lightheadedness, flushing of the face or neck, headache, nausea and vomiting or a fast pulse.

NITROGLYCERIN TRANSDERMAL
Deponit, Minitran Transdermal, Nitro-Dur Transdermal,
Nitrodisc, Transderm-Nitro

THIS MEDICATION IS USED:

To prevent angina attacks.

PROPER USE OF THIS MEDICATION:

 Apply the patch to an area of skin free of hair and not subject to excessive movement. The chest is considered the most appropriate part of the body to use.

 DO NOT cut or tamper with the patch.

Patches can be worn while you bathe or shower.

Before applying a new patch REMOVE the OLD PATCH from your skin.

Change the application site with each patch to avoid skin irritation.

SPECIAL INSTRUCTIONS:

 This medicine may cause lightheadedness. Sit or lie down at the first signs. Avoid sudden changes in posture. Be careful going up and down stairs.

Alcoholic beverages can increase the lightheadedness.

 Proper control of your condition requires you to use this medicine as instructed at the same time every day, DO NOT skip a dose nor stop using the medicine without asking your doctor.

If you miss a dose of this medicine, use it as soon as possible. But, if it is almost time for your next dose, skip the missed dose and go back to your regular dose. DO NOT use a double dose.

DO NOT keep or use outdated medication. Keep all medication out of the reach of children.

POSSIBLE SIDE EFFECTS:

 Be sure to tell your doctor if the following occur: persistent lightheadedness, flushing of the face or neck, headache or a fast pulse.

DIGOXIN
Digitoxin, Lanoxicaps, Lanoxin, Lanoxin Pediatric

THIS MEDICATION IS USED:

To improve heartbeat and rhythm. It is given to improve the strength and efficiency of the heart.

PROPER USE OF THIS MEDICATION:

 This medication should be taken with a glass of water and it can be taken with or without food.

 For the liquid form use the dropper supplied to measure the amount of medicine your doctor has ordered. If you do not fully understand how to use the dropper ask your pharmacist.

DO NOT open the capsule form, swallow it whole.

SPECIAL INSTRUCTIONS:

 Proper control of your condition requires you to take this medicine as instructed at the same time every day, DO NOT skip a dose nor stop taking the medicine without asking your doctor.

Some doctors will want you to check your pulse daily while taking this medicine. If it is different than your usual rate (or less than 60 beats per minute) check with your doctor.

 DO NOT take nonprescription cough/cold or diet products without asking your doctor or pharmacist.

Some nonprescription medications may interfere with the action of this medicine. Avoid taking antacids, antidiarrheals, or bulk forming laxatives within 1 hour of taking this medicine.

 It is important that you advise all of your doctors and dentists that you are taking this medicine before starting other treatments.

If you miss a dose of this medicine, take it as soon as possible. But, if it is almost time for your next dose, skip the missed dose and go back to your regular dose. DO NOT take a double dose.

DO NOT keep or use outdated medication. Keep all medication out of the reach of children.

POSSIBLE SIDE EFFECTS:

Be sure to tell your doctor if the following occur: loss of appetite, nausea and vomiting, diarrhea or slower than normal pulse rate.

NITRATE, ORAL

Dilatrate SR, Duotrate SR, Ismo, Isordil, Isordil Tembids, Isosorbide, Nitro-Bid Plateau, Nitroglycerin, Nitrong, Peritrate, Peritrate SA, Sorbitrate, Sorbitrate SA

THIS MEDICATION IS USED:

To prevent angina attacks.

PROPER USE OF THIS MEDICATION:

 This medicine should be taken on an empty stomach 1 hour before or 2 hours after eating a meal with a glass of water to maximize absorption.

If you are taking the chewable form, it should be chewed well before swallowing.

The controlled release forms should be swallowed whole, NOT crushed or chewed.

SPECIAL INSTRUCTIONS:

The first few doses of this medicine may cause headache or flushing. This is normal and will go away after you take this medicine a few times.

 This medicine may cause lightheadedness. Sit or lie down at the first signs. Avoid sudden changes in posture. Be careful going up and down stairs. Be careful driving or performing hazardous tasks.

Alcoholic beverages can increase the lightheadedness.

 Proper control of your condition requires you to take this medicine as instructed at the same time every day, DO NOT skip a dose nor stop taking the medicine without asking your doctor.

 Store this medicine in a cool dry place, NOT in the refrigerator or medicine cabinet.

If you miss a dose of this medicine, take it as soon as possible. But, if it is almost time for your next dose, skip the missed dose and go back to your regular dose. DO NOT take a double dose.

DO NOT keep or use outdated medication. Keep all medication out of the reach of children.

POSSIBLE SIDE EFFECTS:

 Be sure to tell your doctor if the following occur: persistent lightheadedness, flushing of the face and neck, headache, nausea and vomiting or a fast pulse.

DIPYRIDAMOLE, PERSANTINE

THIS MEDICATION IS USED:

For a number of conditions including reduction of blood clot formation after surgery that repairs or replaces heart valves.

PROPER USE OF THIS MEDICATION:

 Unless your doctor has told you differently, this medicine should be taken on an empty stomach with a glass of water at least 1 hour before or 2 hours after a meal.

If stomach upset occurs, you may take this medicine with food unless told otherwise.

SPECIAL INSTRUCTIONS:

 Proper control of your condition requires you to take this medicine as instructed at the same time every day, DO NOT skip a dose nor stop taking the medicine without asking your doctor.

 If you have a fever or pain, do not take nonprescription aspirin products while taking this medicine without asking your doctor or pharmacist.

 You may experience dizziness, blurred vision or drowsiness from this medicine. If you do, be careful driving or performing hazardous tasks.

If you miss a dose of this medicine, take it as soon as possible. But, if it is almost time for your next dose, skip the missed dose and go back to your regular dose. DO NOT take a double dose.

DO NOT keep or use outdated medication. Keep all medication out of the reach of children.

POSSIBLE SIDE EFFECTS:

 Be sure to tell your doctor if the following occur: dizziness or lightheadedness, flushing, headache or nausea.

CALCIUM CHANNEL BLOCKER

Adalat, Calan, Cardene, Cardene SR, Cardizem, Cardizem CD, Cardizem SR, Diltiazem, Dynacirc, Isoptin, Nifedipine, Norvasc, Plendil, Procardia, Procardia XL, Vascor, Verapamil, Verelan

THIS MEDICATION IS USED:

 For many conditions, including high blood pressure, angina and irregular heartbeat.

PROPER USE OF THIS MEDICATION:

 Some forms of this medication should be taken on an empty stomach with a glass of water, others may be taken without regards to food. If you have not been told which is best, check with your doctor or pharmacist.

 The controlled release forms should be swallowed whole, NOT crushed or chewed.

SPECIAL INSTRUCTIONS:

 This medicine may cause lightheadedness. Sit or lie down at the first signs. Avoid sudden changes in posture. Be careful going up and down stairs. Be careful driving or performing hazardous tasks.

The use of alcohol while taking this medicine may increase the chance of dizziness.

 Proper control of your condition requires you to take this medicine as instructed at the same time every day, DO NOT skip a dose nor stop taking the medicine without asking your doctor.

Since this medicine does not cure but helps to control your condition, you should continue to take it even if you are feeling well.

 DO NOT take nonprescription cough/cold or diet products without asking your doctor or pharmacist.

If you miss a dose of this medicine, take it as soon as possible. But, if it is almost time for your next dose, skip the missed dose and go back to your regular dose. DO NOT take a double dose.

DO NOT keep or use outdated medication. Keep all medication out of the reach of children.

POSSIBLE SIDE EFFECTS:

 Be sure to tell your doctor if the following occur: headache, nausea, swelling of the extremities, unusually slow heartbeat, chest pain, unusual tiredness or difficult breathing.

ANTIHYPERTENSIVE, ALPHA STIMULANT

Aldomet, Catapres, Clonidine, Methyldopa, Tenex, Wytensin

THIS MEDICATION IS USED:

To treat a number of conditions, including high blood pressure.

PROPER USE OF THIS MEDICATION:

This medication should be taken with a glass of water and it can be taken with or without food.

If it upsets your stomach, take it with food.

SPECIAL INSTRUCTIONS:

This medicine may cause you to be drowsy the first few days you take it or when your doctor increases the amount you are taking. If it does, be careful driving or performing hazardous tasks.

This medicine may cause lightheadedness. Sit or lie down at the first signs. Avoid sudden changes in posture. Be careful going up and down stairs.

Alcoholic beverages can increase the drowsiness.

Proper control of your condition requires you to take this medicine as instructed at the same time every day, DO NOT skip a dose nor stop taking the medicine without asking your doctor.

Since this medicine does not cure but helps to control your condition, you should continue to take it even if you are feeling well.

DO NOT take nonprescription cough/cold or diet products without asking your doctor or pharmacist.

If you miss a dose of this medicine, take it as soon as possible. But, if it is almost time for your next dose, skip the missed dose and go back to your regular dose. DO NOT take a double dose.

DO NOT keep or use outdated medication. Keep all medication out of the reach of children.

POSSIBLE SIDE EFFECTS:

 Be sure to tell your doctor if the following occur: changes in moods or dream patterns, nausea, fainting, chest pain, unusual swelling or weight gain or yellow coloration of skin or eyes.

CAPOTEN

THIS MEDICATION IS USED:

 To treat high blood pressure. It is also used to treat congestive heart failure.

PROPER USE OF THIS MEDICATION:

 This medicine should be taken on an empty stomach, one hour before meals.

SPECIAL INSTRUCTIONS:

 This medicine may cause lightheadedness. Sit or lie down at the first signs. Avoid sudden changes in posture. Be careful going up and down stairs. Be careful driving or performing hazardous tasks.

 Proper control of your condition requires you to take this medicine as instructed at the same time every day, DO NOT skip a dose nor stop taking the medicine without asking your doctor.

Since this medicine does not cure but helps to control your condition, you should continue to take it even if you are feeling well.

 You should not use salt substitutes or take nonprescription cough/cold or diet products without asking your doctor or pharmacist.

 If you become pregnant, consult your doctor promptly about switching to a different drug.

If you miss a dose of this medicine, take it as soon as possible. But, if it is almost time for your next dose, skip the missed dose and go back to your regular dose. DO NOT take a double dose.

DO NOT keep or use outdated medicine. Keep this medicine at room temperature, in its original container and out of the reach of children.

POSSIBLE SIDE EFFECTS:

 Be sure to tell your doctor if the following occur: persistent sore throat or fever, swelling of the extremities, eyes, lips, face or tongue, difficult breathing, impaired taste, skin rash, nausea or vomiting.

PROPRANOLOL, PROPRANOLOL LA
Inderal, Inderal LA

THIS MEDICATION IS USED:

 For many conditions, including high blood pressure, angina, irregular heartbeat and prophylaxis of migraine headaches.

PROPER USE OF THIS MEDICATION:

 This medicine can be taken with food or on an empty stomach. However, to maintain the proper amount in the body, it is best that each dose either always be taken with food or always be taken on an empty stomach.

 The controlled release forms should be swallowed whole, NOT crushed or chewed.

The liquid form should be diluted in water or juice using the measuring device provided with your medication.

SPECIAL INSTRUCTIONS:

 This medicine may cause lightheadedness. Sit or lie down at the first signs. Avoid sudden changes in posture. Be careful going up and down stairs. Be careful driving or performing hazardous tasks.

 Proper control of your condition requires you to take this medicine as instructed at the same time every day, DO NOT skip a dose nor stop taking the medicine without asking your doctor.

Since this medicine does not cure but helps to control your condition, you should continue to take it even if you are feeling well.

 DO NOT take nonprescription cough/cold or diet products without asking your doctor or pharmacist.

If you miss a dose of this medicine, take it as soon as possible. But, if it is almost time for your next dose, skip the missed dose and go back to your regular dose. DO NOT take a double dose.

DO NOT keep or use outdated medication. Keep all medication out of the reach of children.

POSSIBLE SIDE EFFECTS:

 Be sure to tell your doctor if the following occur: excessive dizziness or drowsiness, unusually slow pulse, slow irregular heartbeat, difficult breathing, weakness, restlessness, chest pain or mental confusion.

BETA BLOCKER

Atenolol, Blocadren, Cartrol, Corgard, Kerlone, Levatol, Lopressor, Normodyne, Pindolol, Sectral, Tenormin, Timolol, Toprol XL, Trandate, Visken, Zebeta

THIS MEDICATION IS USED:

 For many conditions, including high blood pressure, angina and irregular heartbeat.

PROPER USE OF THIS MEDICATION:

 This medicine can be taken with food or on an empty stomach. However, to maintain the proper amount in the body, it is best that each dose either always be taken with food or always be taken on an empty stomach.

 The controlled release forms should be swallowed whole, NOT crushed or chewed.

SPECIAL INSTRUCTIONS:

 This medicine may cause lightheadedness. Sit or lie down at the first signs. Avoid sudden changes in posture. Be careful going up and down stairs. Be careful driving or performing hazardous tasks.

 Proper control of your condition requires you to take this medicine as instructed at the same time every day, DO NOT skip a dose nor stop taking the medicine without asking your doctor.

Since this medicine does not cure but helps to control your condition, you should continue to take it even if you are feeling well.

 DO NOT take nonprescription cough/cold or diet products without asking your doctor or pharmacist.

If you miss a dose of this medicine, take it as soon as possible. But, if it is almost time for your next dose, skip the missed dose and go back to your regular dose. DO NOT take a double dose.

DO NOT keep or use outdated medication. Keep all medication out of the reach of children.

POSSIBLE SIDE EFFECTS:

 Be sure to tell your doctor if the following occur: excessive dizziness or drowsiness, unusually slow pulse, slow irregular heartbeat, difficult breathing, weakness, restlessness, chest pain or mental confusion.

DIURETIC, THIAZIDE

Aquatensen, Chlorothiazide, Chlorthalidone, Diucardin, Diulo, Diuril, Enduron, Enduronyl, Esidrix, Exna, Hydrex, Hydrochlorothiazide, Hydrodiuril, Hydroflumethiazide, Hydromal, Hydromox, Hygroton, Lozol, Metahydrin, Methyclothiazide, Metolazone, Mykrox, Naturetin, Oretic, Regroton, Renese, Saluron, Trichlormethiazide, Zaroxolyn

THIS MEDICATION IS USED:

To help remove excess fluid and salt, decrease swelling and treat high blood pressure.

PROPER USE OF THIS MEDICATION:

Take this medicine at the same time every day. The best time is in the morning before breakfast.

If stomach upset occurs, you may take this medicine with food unless told otherwise.

Some of the liquid forms require the contents to be shaken well before measuring the dose. Others should be measured using the dropper supplied. If you have any questions on how to measure your dose ask your pharmacist.

SPECIAL INSTRUCTIONS:

Proper control of your condition requires you to take this medicine as instructed at the same time every day, DO NOT skip a dose nor stop taking the medicine without asking your doctor.

Since this medicine does not cure but helps to control your condition, you should continue to take it even if you are feeling well.

This medicine may make your skin more sensitive to sunlight or sunlamps. Ask your pharmacist about a suitable sunblock product (of at least SPF 15) to minimize problems during exposure.

DO NOT take nonprescription cough/cold or diet products without asking your doctor or pharmacist.

If you miss a dose of this medicine, take it as soon as possible. But, if it is almost time for your next dose, skip the missed dose and go back to your regular dose. DO NOT take a double dose.

DO NOT keep or use outdated medication. Keep all medication out of the reach of children.

POSSIBLE SIDE EFFECTS:

 Be sure to tell your doctor if the following occur: persistent sore throat or fever, unusual bleeding, stomach pain, yellow coloration of the eyes or skin, unusual weakness or tiredness, muscle cramps or nausea or vomiting.

ALDACTAZIDE, DYAZIDE
Spironolactone w/Hctz, Triamterene w/Hydrochlorothiazide

THIS MEDICATION IS USED:

To help remove excess fluid and salt, decrease swelling and treat high blood pressure.

PROPER USE OF THIS MEDICATION:

You should take this medicine at the same time every day. The best time is in the morning before breakfast. If stomach upset occurs, you may take this medication with food unless told otherwise.

SPECIAL INSTRUCTIONS:

This medicine may cause lightheadedness. Sit or lie down at the first signs. Avoid sudden changes in posture. Be careful going up and down stairs.

Proper control of your condition requires you to take this medicine as instructed at the same time every day, DO NOT skip a dose nor stop taking the medicine without asking your doctor.

Since this medicine does not cure but helps to control your condition, you should continue to take it even if you are feeling well.

You should NOT use salt substitutes without asking your doctor or pharmacist.

DO NOT take nonprescription cough/cold or diet products without asking your doctor or pharmacist.

This medicine may make your skin more sensitive to sunlight or sunlamps. Ask your pharmacist about a suitable sunblock product (of at least SPF 15) to minimize problems during exposure.

If you miss a dose of this medicine, take it as soon as possible. But, if it is almost time for your next dose, skip the missed dose and go back to your regular dose. DO NOT take a double dose.

DO NOT keep or use outdated medication. Keep all medication out of the reach of children.

POSSIBLE SIDE EFFECTS:

 Be sure to tell your doctor if the following occur: light-headedness, nausea or vomiting or muscle weakness or cramps, sore throat or yellow coloration of the eyes or skin.

DIURETIC, LOOP
Bumex, Furosemide, Lasix

THIS MEDICATION IS USED:

To help remove excess fluid and salt, decrease swelling and treat high blood pressure.

PROPER USE OF THIS MEDICATION:

Take this medicine at the same time every day. The best time is in the morning before breakfast.

If stomach upset occurs, you may take this medicine with food unless told otherwise.

The liquid form should be measured using the measuring device provided with your medication. If you have any questions on how to measure your dose ask your pharmacist.

SPECIAL INSTRUCTIONS:

Proper control of your condition requires you to take this medicine as instructed at the same time every day, DO NOT skip a dose nor stop taking the medicine without asking your doctor.

Since this medicine does not cure but helps to control your condition, you should continue to take it even if you are feeling well.

This medicine may make your skin more sensitive to sunlight or sunlamps. Ask your pharmacist about a suitable sunblock product (of at least SPF 15) to minimize problems during exposure.

DO NOT take nonprescription cough/cold or diet products without asking your doctor or pharmacist.

If you miss a dose of this medicine, take it as soon as possible. But, if it is almost time for your next dose, skip the missed dose and go back to your regular dose. DO NOT take a double dose.

DO NOT keep or use outdated medication. Keep all medication out of the reach of children.

POSSIBLE SIDE EFFECTS:

 Be sure to tell your doctor if the following occur: persistent sore throat or fever, unusual bleeding, stomach pain, yellow coloration of the eyes or skin, unusual weakness or tiredness, muscle cramps or nausea or vomiting.

POTASSIUM, SOLID

K-Dur, K-Norm, K-Tab, Kaon CL, Klor-Con, Klotrix Tablet, Micro-K Extencaps, Potassium Gluconate, Slow K, Ten K

THIS MEDICATION IS USED:

As a potassium supplement.

PROPER USE OF THIS MEDICATION:

Take this medication with food and a glass of water to help avoid upsetting your stomach.

Capsule forms of this medication can be swallowed whole or opened up and the contents mixed with food.

Some tablets should be swallowed whole. DO NOT crush, chew or grind them up.

Other tablets can be crushed, broken and sprinkled on food before taking them. If you are not sure whether the medication you are taking can or cannot be crushed, ask your pharmacist.

SPECIAL INSTRUCTIONS:

You should NOT use salt substitutes without asking your doctor or pharmacist. These products also contain potassium.

It is recommended that you drink lots of fluids while taking this medication.

It is important that you take this medicine exactly as your doctor has instructed.

If you miss a dose of this medicine, take it as soon as possible. But, if it is almost time for your next dose, skip the missed dose and go back to your regular dose. DO NOT take a double dose.

DO NOT keep or use outdated medication. Keep all medication out of the reach of children.

POSSIBLE SIDE EFFECTS:

 Be sure to tell your doctor if the following occur: irregular heartbeat, unusual tiredness, difficult breathing, mental confusion, numbness or tingling in the extremities, severe vomiting, abdominal pain or black tarry stools.

ANTICOAGULANT
Coumadin, Dicumarol

THIS MEDICATION IS USED:

To help prevent blood clots from forming in the blood vessels.

PROPER USE OF THIS MEDICATION:

 This medication should be taken with a glass of water and it can be taken with or without food.

SPECIAL INSTRUCTIONS:

 Proper control of your condition requires you to take this medicine as instructed at the same time every day, DO NOT skip a dose nor stop taking the medicine without asking your doctor.

 DO NOT take nonprescription medications or vitamins (i.e. aspirin, antacids and laxatives) without telling your doctor.

 Since adequate but not excessive intake of vitamin K is required, you should eat a well-balanced diet and not experiment with fad diets or weight reduction schemes without consulting your doctor.

Periodic blood tests are necessary in order for your doctor to prescribe the correct dose.

 It is recommended that alcohol intake be minimized while on this medication.

If you miss a dose of this medicine, take it as soon as possible. But, if it is almost time for your next dose, skip the missed dose and go back to your regular dose. DO NOT take a double dose.

DO NOT keep or use outdated medication. Keep all medication out of the reach of children.

POSSIBLE SIDE EFFECTS:

 Be sure to tell your doctor if the following occur: excessive or unusual bleeding or bruising, persistent headache, fever, sore throat, backache or stomach pain, yellow coloration of the eyes or skin, swelling of the extremities, mouth sores, persistent constipation or diarrhea and darkened or bloody urine or stools.

ANTISPASMODIC

Anaspaz, Bentyl, Cystospaz, Dicyclomine, Donnatal, Levsin, Levsin/Phenobarbital, Pro-Banthine, Propantheline

THIS MEDICATION IS USED:

To treat stomach and intestinal disorders.

PROPER USE OF THIS MEDICATION:

 This medication works best when taken 30 to 60 minutes before meals and at bedtime.

If this medication upsets your stomach it can be taken with food.

 Antacids may inhibit the absorption of some forms of this medication and should not be taken within 2 hours of a dose.

 The controlled release forms should be swallowed whole, NOT crushed or chewed.

If you are taking the liquid form, there are special measuring devices available to measure your dose, ask your pharmacist if you want one.

SPECIAL INSTRUCTIONS:

 You may experience dizziness, blurred vision or drowsiness from this medicine. If you do, be careful driving or performing hazardous tasks.

 Alcoholic beverages can increase the drowsiness.

If your mouth becomes dry, you may suck on hard candy, chew gum or use a saliva substitute.

 If taken for a few days, you may experience some constipation. You should increase the amount of bulk in your diet (bran, psyllium, and fresh fruits) and drink fluids.

If you miss a dose of this medicine, take it as soon as possible. But, if it is almost time for your next dose, skip the missed dose and go back to your regular dose. DO NOT take a double dose.

DO NOT keep or use outdated medication. Keep all medication out of the reach of children.

POSSIBLE SIDE EFFECTS:

 Be sure to tell your doctor if the following occur: blurred vision or eye pain, dry mouth, difficult urination, constipation, difficulty in speaking or persistent sore throat or fever.

HISTAMINE – 2 BLOCKER
Axid, Tagamet, Zantac

THIS MEDICATION IS USED:

To treat a number of conditions, including ulcers and other diseases in which the stomach produces too much acid.

PROPER USE OF THIS MEDICATION:

The best time to take this medicine is before meals to reduce the increased stomach acid that occurs after meals. The bedtime dose does not need to be taken with food.

 If you are using antacids, they should be taken 1 hour before or after this medicine.

If you are taking the liquid form, there are special measuring devices available, ask your pharmacist if you want one.

SPECIAL INSTRUCTIONS:

 Proper control of your condition requires you to take this medicine as instructed at the same time every day, DO NOT skip a dose nor stop taking the medicine without asking your doctor.

You should continue to take this medicine even if you are feeling better to help prevent future stomach pain.

 You may experience dizziness, blurred vision or drowsiness from this medicine. If you do, be careful driving or performing hazardous tasks.

If you miss a dose of this medicine, take it as soon as possible. But, if it is almost time for your next dose, skip the missed dose and go back to your regular dose. DO NOT take a double dose.

DO NOT keep or use outdated medication. Keep all medication out of the reach of children.

POSSIBLE SIDE EFFECTS:

 Be sure to tell your doctor if the following occur: persistent dizziness or headache, skin rash, confusion or black tarry stools.

CARAFATE, SUCRALFATE

THIS MEDICATION IS USED:

To treat ulcers.

PROPER USE OF THIS MEDICATION:

 This medicine should be taken on an empty stomach at least 1 hour before or 2 hours after meals and at bedtime with a glass of water.

 If your doctor has told you to take antacids while on this medicine, they may be taken within 30 minutes before or after this medicine.

These tablets may be split in two for easier swallowing.

SPECIAL INSTRUCTIONS:

 Proper control of your condition requires you to take this medicine as instructed at the same time every day, DO NOT skip a dose nor stop taking the medicine without asking your doctor.

If you miss a dose of this medicine, take it as soon as possible. But, if it is almost time for your next dose, skip the missed dose and go back to your regular dose. DO NOT take a double dose.

DO NOT keep or use outdated medication. Keep all medication out of the reach of children.

POSSIBLE SIDE EFFECTS:

 Be sure to tell your doctor if the following occur: skin rash, constipation, dry mouth, nausea or diarrhea.

METOCLOPRAMIDE, REGLAN

THIS MEDICATION IS USED:

To treat the symptoms of nausea, vomiting, persistent fullness after meals and loss of appetite.

PROPER USE OF THIS MEDICATION:

 This medicine is best taken 30 minutes before a meal and at bedtime with a full glass of water.

 If you are taking the liquid form, there are special measuring devices available to measure your dose, ask your pharmacist if you want one.

SPECIAL INSTRUCTIONS:

 You may experience dizziness, blurred vision or drowsiness from this medicine. If you do, be careful driving or performing hazardous tasks.

Alcoholic beverages can increase the drowsiness.

 Proper control of your condition requires you to take this medicine as instructed at the same time every day, DO NOT skip a dose nor stop taking the medicine without asking your doctor.

If you miss a dose of this medicine, take it as soon as possible. But, if it is almost time for your next dose, skip the missed dose and go back to your regular dose. DO NOT take a double dose.

DO NOT keep or use outdated medication. Keep all medication out of the reach of children.

POSSIBLE SIDE EFFECTS:

 Be sure to tell your doctor if the following occur: drowsiness, dizziness, restlessness, unusual tiredness or weakness, uncontrolled trembling of the extremities or movements of the tongue, jerky movements of the head, face or mouth, muscle spasms of the neck or back or a shuffling walk.

BENZODIAZEPINE

Ativan, Centrax, Chlordiazepoxide, Clorazepate, Diazepam,
Klonopin, Libritabs, Librium, Lorazepam, Oxazepam, Paxipam,
Prazepam, Serax, Tranxene, Valium, Valrelease, Xanax

THIS MEDICATION IS USED:

To relieve anxiety and tension, relax muscles or relieve muscle spasms. Some are used to treat certain convulsive disorders.

PROPER USE OF THIS MEDICATION:

This medication should be taken with a glass of water and it can be taken with or without food.

The controlled release forms should be swallowed whole, NOT crushed or chewed.

Some liquid forms, should be diluted in water or juice using the measuring device provided with your medication.

SPECIAL INSTRUCTIONS:

You may experience dizziness, blurred vision or drowsiness from this medicine. If you do, be careful driving or performing hazardous tasks.

Alcoholic beverages can increase the drowsiness.

It is important that you take this medicine exactly as your doctor has instructed. DO NOT increase nor stop taking this medicine without consulting your doctor.

If you miss a dose of this medicine, take it as soon as possible. But, if it is almost time for your next dose, skip the missed dose and go back to your regular dose. DO NOT take a double dose.

DO NOT keep or use outdated medication. Keep all medication out of the reach of children.

POSSIBLE SIDE EFFECTS:

Be sure to tell your doctor if the following occur: persistent fever or sore throat, mouth sores, difficulty breathing, irregular heartbeat, yellow coloration of the skin or eyes, excessive confusion or excitement.

TRICYCLIC ANTIDEPRESSANT

Amitriptyline, Amoxapine, Asendin, Aventyl, Desipramine, Doxepin, Elavil, Endep, Imipramine, Ludiomil, Norpramin, Nortriptyline, Pamelor, Pertofrane, Sinequan, Surmontil, Tofranil, Tofranil-PM, Vivactil

THIS MEDICATION IS USED:

To relieve depression.

PROPER USE OF THIS MEDICATION:

 Take this medicine with a glass of water. If it upsets your stomach you may take it with food.

 Some liquid forms, should be diluted in water or juice using the measuring device provided with your medication. If you do not understand how to measure the dose ask your pharmacist.

SPECIAL INSTRUCTIONS:

 You may experience dizziness, blurred vision or drowsiness from this medicine. Be careful driving or performing hazardous tasks.

 Alcoholic beverages can increase the drowsiness.

This medicine may cause lightheadedness. Sit or lie down at the first signs. Avoid sudden changes in posture. Be careful going up and down stairs.

 DO NOT take nonprescription cough/cold, hay fever, diet or sleep aid products without asking your doctor or pharmacist.

It may take several weeks before the full effects of this medicine are noticed. DO NOT change the amount of medicine taken nor stop taking it without consulting your doctor.

If your mouth becomes dry, you may suck on hard candy, chew gum or use a saliva substitute.

 If taken for a few days, you may experience some constipation. You should increase the amount of bulk in your diet (bran, psyllium, and fresh fruits) and drink lots of fluids.

This medicine may make your skin more sensitive to sunlight or sunlamps. Ask your pharmacist about a suitable sunblock product (of at least SPF 15) to minimize problems during exposure.

If you miss a dose of this medicine, take it as soon as possible. But, if it is almost time for your next dose, skip the missed dose and go back to your regular dose. DO NOT take a double dose.

DO NOT keep or use outdated medication. Keep all medication out of the reach of children.

POSSIBLE SIDE EFFECTS:

Be sure to tell your doctor if the following occur: blurred vision or eye pain, nervousness or confusion, irregular heartbeat or pulse, fainting spells, difficulty getting to sleep or urinating, severe drowsiness, troubled breathing, high fever or hallucinations.

TRAZODONE, DESYREL

THIS MEDICATION IS USED:

To treat depression.

PROPER USE OF THIS MEDICATION:

 This medication should be taken after meals or a light snack to maximize absorption.

SPECIAL INSTRUCTIONS:

 You may experience dizziness, blurred vision or drowsiness from this medicine. If you do, be careful driving or performing hazardous tasks.

Alcoholic beverages can increase the drowsiness.

 This medicine may cause lightheadedness. Sit or lie down at the first signs. Avoid sudden changes in posture. Be careful going up and down stairs.

 DO NOT take nonprescription cough/cold, hay fever, diet or sleep aid products without asking your doctor or pharmacist.

 It may take several weeks before the full effects of this medicine are noticed. DO NOT change the amount of medicine taken nor stop taking it without consulting your doctor.

If you miss a dose of this medicine, take it as soon as possible. But, if it is almost time for your next dose, skip the missed dose and go back to your regular dose. DO NOT take a double dose.

DO NOT keep or use outdated medication. Keep all medication out of the reach of children.

POSSIBLE SIDE EFFECTS:

 Be sure to tell your doctor if the following occur: blurred vision or eye pain, nervousness or confusion, irregular heartbeat or pulse, fainting spells, difficulty getting to sleep or urinating, severe drowsiness, troubled breathing, high fever, hallucinations, excessive sweating or seizures.

ANTIPSYCHOTIC

Chlorpromazine, Chlorpromazine Concentrate, Compazine, Fluphenazine, Haldol, Haldol Concentrate, Haloperidol, Haloperidol Concentrate, Mellaril, Mellaril-S, Navane, Navane Concentrate, Permitil, Permitil Concentrate, Perphenazine, Prochlorperazine, Prolixin, Serentil, Sparine, Stelazine, Stelazine Concentrate, Thioridazine, Thioridazine Concentrate, Thiothixene, Thiothixene Concentrate, Thorazine, Thorazine Concentrate, Thorazine Spansule, Tindal, Trifluoperazine, Trifluoperazine Concentrate, Trilafon, Trilafon Concentrate

THIS MEDICATION IS USED:

To relieve emotional problems, such as anxiety, agitation, depressed mood and tension.

PROPER USE OF THIS MEDICATION:

Take this medicine with a glass of water. If it upsets your stomach you may take it with food.

DO NOT take within 1-2 hours of an antacid.

Some capsule forms of this medication can be swallowed whole or opened up and the contents mixed with food.

Other controlled release forms should be swallowed whole, NOT crushed, chewed or broken. If you are not sure which is your type of medication, ask your pharmacist.

Some liquid forms, should be diluted in water or juice using the measuring device provided with your medication. If you do not understand how to measure your dose, ask your pharmacist.

SPECIAL INSTRUCTIONS:

You may experience dizziness, blurred vision or drowsiness from this medicine. If you do, be careful driving or performing hazardous tasks.

Alcoholic beverages can increase the drowsiness.

This medicine may cause lightheadedness. Sit or lie down at the first signs. Avoid sudden changes in posture. Be careful going up and down stairs.

It may take several weeks before the full effects of this medicine are noticed. DO NOT change the amount of medicine taken nor stop taking it without consulting your doctor.

 DO NOT take nonprescription cough/cold, hay fever, antacids, antidiarrheals, diet or sleep aid products without asking your doctor or pharmacist.

If your mouth becomes dry, you may suck on hard candy, chew gum or use a saliva substitute.

 It is recommended that you drink lots of fluids while taking this medication.

 This medicine may make your skin more sensitive to sunlight or sunlamps. Ask your pharmacist about a suitable sunblock product (of at least SPF 15) to minimize problems during exposure.

If you miss a dose of this medicine, take it as soon as possible. But, if it is almost time for your next dose, skip the missed dose and go back to your regular dose. DO NOT take a double dose.

DO NOT keep or use outdated medication. Keep all medication out of the reach of children.

POSSIBLE SIDE EFFECTS:

 Be sure to tell your doctor if the following occur: persistent sore throat or fever, blurred vision, yellow coloration of the eyes or skin, uncontrollable trembling of the extremities or movement of the tongue, jerky movements of the head, face or mouth or shuffling walk.

ANTIDYSKINETIC
Akineton, Artane, Benztropine Mesylate,
Cogentin, Trihexyphenidyl

THIS MEDICATION IS USED:

To treat Parkinson's disease and drug-induced parkinsonism.

PROPER USE OF THIS MEDICATION:

 This medication should be taken with a glass of water and it can be taken with or without food.

 The controlled release forms should be swallowed whole, NOT crushed or chewed.

If you are taking the liquid form, there are special measuring devices available to measure your dose, ask your pharmacist if you want one.

SPECIAL INSTRUCTIONS:

 You may experience dizziness, blurred vision or drowsiness from this medicine. If you do, be careful driving or performing hazardous tasks.

 Alcoholic beverages can increase the drowsiness.

If your mouth becomes dry, you may suck on hard candy, chew gum or use a saliva substitute.

 If taken for a few days, you may experience some constipation. You should increase the amount of bulk in your diet (bran, psyllium, and fresh fruits) and drink lots of fluids.

If you miss a dose of this medicine, take it as soon as possible. But, if it is almost time for your next dose, skip the missed dose and go back to your regular dose. DO NOT take a double dose.

DO NOT keep or use outdated medication. Keep all medication out of the reach of children.

POSSIBLE SIDE EFFECTS:

 Be sure to tell your doctor if the following occur: blurred vision or eye pain, dry mouth, difficult urination, constipation, rapid heartbeat, confusion or skin rash.

BENZODIAZEPINE, HYPNOTIC

Dalmane, Doral, Flurazepam, Halcion,
Prosom, Restoril, Temazepam

THIS MEDICATION IS USED:

To treat insomnia.

PROPER USE OF THIS MEDICATION:

 You should take this medicine with a glass of water before bedtime. If it upsets your stomach you may take it with food.

SPECIAL INSTRUCTIONS:

 If you experience any next day drowsiness or "hangover" from this medicine, DO NOT drive a car or perform hazardous tasks.

 Alcoholic beverages can increase the drowsiness.

It is important that you take this medicine exactly as your doctor has instructed. DO NOT increase your dose nor take longer than 7-10 days without consulting your doctor.

 If you experience unusual thoughts or behavior while taking this medicine, talk to your doctor.

Some people experience disturbed sleep for 1 or 2 days after discontinuing this medication. This should go away in a few days. If it continues contact your doctor.

DO NOT take any nonprescription sleep aid medicine without first asking your doctor or pharmacist.

Tell your doctor if you are pregnant, plan to become pregnant or are breastfeeding.

DO NOT keep or use outdated medication. Keep all medication out of the reach of children.

POSSIBLE SIDE EFFECTS:

 Be sure to tell your doctor if the following occur: persistent fever or sore throat, mouth sores, difficulty breathing, irregular heartbeat, yellow coloration of the skin or eyes, excessive confusion or excitement.

HYDANTOIN ANTICONVULSANT

Dilantin, Mephenytoin, Mesantoin, Peganone

THIS MEDICATION IS USED:

To control convulsions and seizures.

PROPER USE OF THIS MEDICATION:

 Take this medicine with a glass of water. If it upsets your stomach you may take it with food.

 If you are taking the liquid form, the contents should be shaken vigorously just before measuring the dose. There are special measuring devices available, ask your pharmacist if you want one.

 If you are taking the chewable form, it should be chewed well before swallowing.

SPECIAL INSTRUCTIONS:

 You may experience dizziness, blurred vision or drowsiness from this medicine. If you do, be careful driving or performing hazardous tasks.

Alcoholic beverages can increase the drowsiness.

 Proper control of your condition requires you to take this medicine as instructed at the same time every day, DO NOT skip a dose nor stop taking the medicine without asking your doctor.

 Maintain good oral hygiene (regular brushing and flossing) while taking this medicine. Call your doctor if your gums become tender or swollen.

If you miss a dose of this medicine, take it as soon as possible. But, if it is almost time for your next dose, skip the missed dose and go back to your regular dose. DO NOT take a double dose.

DO NOT keep or use outdated medication. Keep all medication out of the reach of children.

POSSIBLE SIDE EFFECTS:

 Be sure to tell your doctor if the following occur: bleeding, swollen or tender gums, slurred speech, uncontrolled eye movement, staggered walk, yellow coloration of the eyes or skin, unusual bleeding or bruising or persistent sore throat or fever.

THYROID

Armour Thyroid, Cytomel, L-Thyroxine Sodium, Levo-T,
Levothroid, Levothyroxine, Levoxine, Synthroid, Thyroid, Thyrolar

THIS MEDICATION IS USED:

To treat conditions when the body is not producing enough thyroid hormone.

PROPER USE OF THIS MEDICATION:

Unless your doctor has told you differently, this medicine should be taken on an empty stomach with a glass of water before breakfast.

SPECIAL INSTRUCTIONS:

Proper control of your condition requires you to take this medicine as instructed at the same time every day, DO NOT skip a dose nor stop taking the medicine without asking your doctor.

Since this medicine does not cure but helps to control your condition, you should continue to take it even if you are feeling well.

DO NOT take nonprescription cough/cold or diet products without asking your doctor or pharmacist.

If you miss a dose of this medicine, take it as soon as possible. But, if it is almost time for your next dose, skip the missed dose and go back to your regular dose. DO NOT take a double dose.

DO NOT keep or use outdated medication. Keep all medication out of the reach of children.

POSSIBLE SIDE EFFECTS:

Be sure to tell your doctor if the following occur: nervousness, irritability, diarrhea, heat intolerance, excessive sweating, increased pulse rate, heart palpitations, prolonged headache or fever or difficult breathing.

ANTIDIARRHEAL, ANTIPERASTALTIC
Diphenoxylate w/Atropine, Lomotil

THIS MEDICATION IS USED:
To treat diarrhea.

PROPER USE OF THIS MEDICATION:

 Take this medicine with a glass of water. If it upsets your stomach you may take it with food.

 For the liquid form, use the measuring device provided with your medication to measure your dose. If you need assistance in understanding how to use the device, ask your pharmacist.

SPECIAL INSTRUCTIONS:

If your diarrhea does not stop after a few days or if you develop a high fever, call your doctor.

 You may experience dizziness, blurred vision or drowsiness from this medicine. If you do, be careful driving or performing hazardous tasks.

 Alcoholic beverages can increase drowsiness.

If your mouth becomes dry, you may suck on hard candy, chew gum or use a saliva substitute.

 You should drink extra fluids each day to help replace the fluid your body has lost due to the diarrhea.

If you miss a dose of this medicine, take it as soon as possible. But, if it is almost time for your next dose, skip the missed dose and go back to your regular dose. DO NOT take a double dose.

DO NOT keep or use outdated medication. Keep all medication out of the reach of children.

POSSIBLE SIDE EFFECTS:

 Be sure to tell your doctor if the following occur: nausea or vomiting, blurred vision, shallow breathing, unusual excitement or depression or prolonged fever or eye pain.

ALLOPURINOL
Lopurin, Zyloprim

THIS MEDICATION IS USED:

To treat gout and other conditions in which the body has high levels of uric acid.

PROPER USE OF THIS MEDICATION:

 Take this medicine with a glass of water. If it upsets your stomach you may take it with food.

SPECIAL INSTRUCTIONS:

 It is recommended that you drink lots of fluids while you are taking this medication. This will help prevent kidney stones.

 You may experience dizziness, blurred vision or drowsiness from this medicine. If you do, be careful driving or performing hazardous tasks.

Alcoholic beverages can increase drowsiness.

 Proper control of your condition requires you to take this medicine as instructed at the same time every day, DO NOT skip a dose nor stop taking the medicine without asking your doctor.

 Tell your doctor immediately if you develop a skin rash or swelling of the lips or mouth or notice blood in your urine.

If you miss a dose of this medicine, take it as soon as possible. But, if it is almost time for your next dose, skip the missed dose and go back to your regular dose. DO NOT take a double dose.

DO NOT keep or use outdated medication. Keep all medication out of the reach of children.

POSSIBLE SIDE EFFECTS:

 Be sure to tell your doctor if the following occur: skin rash, hives or itching, painful urination, blood in the urine, irritation of the eyes, swelling of the lips or mouth, diarrhea, nausea or vomiting, persistent sore throat or fever or unusual bleeding or bruising.

KWELL
Kwell Shampoo, Scabene, Scabene Shampoo

THIS MEDICATION IS USED:

To treat head lice, crab lice, and their eggs. The cream and lotion forms are used to treat scabies (mites).

PROPER USE OF THIS MEDICATION:

 This medicine is for EXTERNAL USE ONLY! DO NOT apply to the face. If you get some into your eyes, flush thoroughly with water.

SHAMPOO INSTRUCTIONS

 Apply a sufficient amount to thoroughly cover the dry hair.

Work the shampoo into the hair and allow it to remain there for 4 minutes.

Add small amounts of water to form a lather.

Rinse hair thoroughly and dry with a clean towel.

When hair is dry, comb it with a fine tooth comb to remove any remaining nits (eggs) or nit shells.

DO NOT use as a regular shampoo.

Retreatment is usually not necessary, unless you detect living lice after 7 days.

 Contact your doctor if you feel retreatment is necessary.

TOPICAL APPLICATION

Take a warm bath or shower before using this medication. Make sure the skin is dry before applying this medication.

 Apply a thin layer of medication to the skin, from the neck down, and rub in thoroughly.

Medication should be left on for 8 - 12 hours, then removed completely by washing.

Two ounces is usually a sufficient amount to cover the adult body.

One application is usually curative. Contact your doctor if you feel retreatment is necessary.

SPECIAL INSTRUCTIONS:

 To help prevent reinfestation and the spread of lice to other people, all clothes, bed linen and towels should be washed in very hot water.

Sexual partners should be treated at the same time to help prevent reinfestation.

DO NOT apply to open wounds or sores.

DO NOT use to prevent an infestation.

DO NOT keep or use outdated medication. Keep all medication out of the reach of children.

In case of accidental ingestion contact your poison control center immediately.

POSSIBLE SIDE EFFECTS:

 Be sure to tell your doctor if the following occur: irritation of the skin or scalp that was not present before treatment.

TOPICAL ANTIFUNGAL

Exelderm, Halotex, Loprox, Miconazole, Monistat-Derm, Naftin, Nizoral Cream, Oxistat, Spectazole

THIS MEDICATION IS USED:

To treat certain fungal infections of the skin.

PROPER USE OF THIS MEDICINE:

This product is for EXTERNAL USE ONLY.

Wash your hands before and after using this medicine.

Cleanse the skin area with soap and water and pat dry each time you are ready to apply the medicine, unless otherwise directed by your doctor.

Apply a small amount of the medication to the affected area and spread lightly.

Only the medicine that is actually touching the skin will work. A thick layer is not more effective than a thin layer.

DO NOT bandage the area unless directed by your doctor.

If your medication is a lotion or a suspension SHAKE the container well before applying.

If your medication is an aerosol spray, SHAKE the container well before applying and hold the container straight up, about 6-8 inches from the affected skin area and spray for 2-3 seconds.

SPECIAL INSTRUCTIONS:

DO NOT use this medication in your eyes.

DO NOT apply any other creams, lotions or cosmetics on top of or beneath this medication.

It is important that you use this medicine exactly as your doctor has instructed.

Use this medication for the full treatment time prescribed by your doctor, even if the symptoms have improved. If improvement does not occur within 4 weeks, you should notify your doctor.

Call your doctor if the condition persists or becomes worse, or if you have a constant burning or itching that was not present before you started this medication.

If you miss a dose of this medicine, use it as soon as possible. But, if it is almost time for your next dose, skip the missed dose and go back to your regular dose. DO NOT use a double dose.

DO NOT keep or use outdated medication. Keep all medication out of the reach of children.

In case of accidental ingestion, call your doctor or poison control center immediately.

POSSIBLE SIDE EFFECTS:

 Be sure to tell your doctor if the following occur: skin rash, hives, blistering, swelling, itching, burning, redness or other signs of skin irritation.

ZOVIRAX

THIS MEDICATION IS USED:

To treat symptoms of herpes virus infections of the skin, mouth and genitals (sex organs). It is also used for the acute treatment of chicken pox and shingles.

PROPER USE OF THIS MEDICATION:

CAPSULES AND ORAL SUSPENSION

This medication should be taken with a glass of water and it can be taken with or without food.

If it upsets your stomach take it with food.

Shake the contents of the suspension well just before measuring the dose. There are special measuring devices available, ask your pharmacist if you want one.

OINTMENT

Is best to apply as soon as symptoms of herpes begin to appear (pain, burning, or blisters).

It should be applied every 3 hours (6 times per day) for at least 7 days unless otherwise instructed by your doctor.

Be sure the ointment fully covers all the herpes sores. Use a finger cot to prevent the spread of infection to other parts of your body and to other people.

Discard the finger cot after applying the medication.

DO NOT use this ointment in your eyes.

SPECIAL INSTRUCTIONS:

It is important that you take or use this medicine exactly as your doctor has instructed.

If your symptoms do not improve within a few days or if they become worse, contact your doctor.

You should tell your doctor if you become pregnant or if you intend to become pregnant while taking this medication.

The area affected by the herpes virus should be kept as clean and dry as possible. Be sure to wear loose fitting clothing while sores and blisters are present to prevent irritation.

REMEMBER, this medication will NOT keep you from spreading herpes to others. Therefore, it is best to avoid any sexual activity or contact if either you or your partner has symptoms of herpes.

If you miss a dose of this medicine, take or use it as soon as possible. But, if it is almost time for your next dose, skip the missed dose and go back to your regular dose. DO NOT take or use a double dose.

DO NOT keep or use outdated medication. Keep all medication out of the reach of children.

In case of accidental ingestion, call your doctor or poison control center immediately.

POSSIBLE SIDE EFFECTS:

Be sure to tell your doctor if the following occur: joint pain, persistent or severe headache, dizziness, or, nausea, vomiting or diarrhea.

NICORETTE

THIS MEDICATION IS USED:

 As a temporary aid to help stop smoking.

PROPER USE OF THIS MEDICATION:

 This medicine is a chewing gum, DO NOT swallow it whole. Chew it slowly until you taste it or feel a slight tingling in your mouth.

As soon as you get the taste of the gum, stop chewing and hold it between the cheek and gum.

After the taste or tingling is almost gone, slowly chew the gum again and repeat the process (usually 30 minutes per piece of gum).

SPECIAL INSTRUCTIONS:

Whenever you feel the urge to smoke, begin to chew 1 piece of gum slowly according to instructions.

 Usually 10 or less pieces of gum per day are enough to control the urge to smoke. If more are needed you should NOT chew more than 30 per day.

Chewing fast will release the nicotine quickly, leading to effects similar to oversmoking.

Gradually reduce the number of pieces of gum you chew each day as your urge to smoke fades.

DO NOT stop using the gum until your craving is satisfied with 1 or 2 pieces a day. However, DO NOT use the gum for more than 6 months without discussing it with your doctor.

 There are more detailed instructions on the proper use of Nicorette along with other patient information to help you stop smoking, ask your doctor or pharmacist for it.

DO NOT drink liquids while chewing Nicorette.

Nicorette itself will NOT cure your smoking habit. The best method is to internalize your desire to be a non-smoker. Nicorette will help offset your cravings for nicotine while quitting.

Nicorette is intended to be an aid to participation in a behavioral modification program. There are a number of "quitters" programs available, ask your doctor or pharmacist for information about them.

You must be committed to quit smoking or Nicorette WILL NOT work.

For Nicorette to work you must use it exactly as directed. DO NOT smoke while you are using it as this can lead to side effects.

Keep Nicorette in its original packaging at room temperature until you are ready to use it.

DO NOT keep or use outdated medication. Keep all medication out of the reach of children.

POSSIBLE SIDE EFFECTS:

 Be sure to tell your doctor if the following occur: sore mouth, rapid heart beat or nausea.

SINEMET

THIS MEDICATION IS USED:

To treat Parkinson's disease.

PROPER USE OF THIS MEDICATION:

 This medicine may be taken with or without food. If it upsets your stomach, take it with food.

 The controlled release forms should be swallowed whole, NOT crushed or chewed.

SPECIAL INSTRUCTIONS:

 You may experience dizziness, blurred vision or drowsiness from this medicine. If you do, be careful driving or performing hazardous tasks.

Alcoholic beverages can increase the drowsiness.

 This medicine may cause lightheadedness. Sit or lie down at the first signs. Avoid sudden changes in posture. Be careful going up and down stairs.

It may take several weeks before the full effects of this medicine are noticed. DO NOT change the amount of medicine taken nor stop taking it without consulting your doctor.

 DO NOT take vitamins containing Vitamin B-6 (pyridoxine) while taking this medication, unless prescribed by your doctor.

If you miss a dose of this medicine, take it as soon as possible. But, if it is almost time for your next dose, skip the missed dose and go back to your regular dose. DO NOT take a double dose.

DO NOT keep or use outdated medication. Keep all medication out of the reach of children.

POSSIBLE SIDE EFFECTS:

Be sure to tell your doctor if the following occur: severe or persistent nausea or vomiting, fainting spells or unusual body movements, changes in mood or nightmares, irregular heartbeat or difficult urination.

HYDROXYZINE
Atarax, Vistaril

THIS MEDICATION IS USED:

To relieve itchiness due to skin rashes and to relieve anxiety and tension.

PROPER USE OF THIS MEDICATION:

Take this medicine with a glass of water. If it upsets your stomach you may take it with food.

Some of the liquid forms require the contents to be shaken well just before measuring the dose. There are special measuring devices available, ask your pharmacist if you want one.

SPECIAL INSTRUCTIONS:

You may experience dizziness, blurred vision or drowsiness from this medicine. If you do, be careful driving or performing hazardous tasks.

Alcoholic beverages can increase the drowsiness.

If your mouth becomes dry, you may suck on hard candy, chew gum or use a saliva substitute.

You should NOT take nonprescription cough/cold products without asking your doctor or pharmacist.

If you miss a dose of this medicine, take it as soon as possible. But, if it is almost time for your next dose, skip the missed dose and go back to your regular dosing schedule. DO NOT take a double dose.

DO NOT keep or use outdated medication. Keep all medication out of the reach of children.

POSSIBLE SIDE EFFECTS:

Be sure to tell your doctor if the following occur: drowsiness, dryness of mouth, dizziness, wheezing, difficulty in breathing, or chest tightness.

ANTIHISTAMINE & DECONGESTANT

Carbodec, Carbodec TR, Cardec S, Comhist, Comhist LA, Deconamine, Dexophed, Disobrom, Fedahist Gyrocaps, Histalet, Histatan Pediatric, Naldecon, Nolamine, Novafed A, Ornade, Phenergan VC, Polyhistine-D, Polyhistine-D Pediatric, Promethazine VC, R-Tannamine Pediatric, R-Tannate Pediatric, Rondec, Rondec Oral Drops, Rondec-TR, Rutuss II, Rynatan, Rynatan Pediatric, Tavist-D, Tri-Phen-Chlor, Tri-Tannate Pediatric, Triaminic Oral Drops, Trinalin Repetabs

THIS MEDICATION IS USED:

To relieve the runny nose, watery eyes, sneezing and stuffiness of colds and hay fever.

PROPER USE OF THIS MEDICATION:

 Take this medicine with a glass of water. If it upsets your stomach you may take it with food.

 Some of the liquid forms require the contents to be shaken well just before measuring the dose. There are special measuring devices available, ask your pharmacist if you want one.

 The pellet and controlled release forms should be swallowed whole, NOT crushed or chewed.

SPECIAL INSTRUCTIONS:

 You may experience dizziness, blurred vision or drowsiness from this medicine. If you do, be careful driving or performing hazardous tasks.

 Alcoholic beverages can increase the drowsiness.

If your mouth becomes dry, you may suck on hard candy, chew gum or use a saliva substitute.

 You should NOT take nonprescription cough/cold products without asking your doctor or pharmacist.

 This medicine may make your skin more sensitive to sunlight or sunlamps. Ask your pharmacist about a suitable sunblock product (of at least SPF 15) to minimize problems during exposure.

If you miss a dose of this medicine, take it as soon as possible. But, if it is almost time for your next dose, skip the missed dose and go back to your regular dose. DO NOT take a double dose.

DO NOT keep or use outdated medication. Keep all medication out of the reach of children.

POSSIBLE SIDE EFFECTS:

Be sure to tell your doctor if the following occur: drowsiness, blurred vision, dry mouth, headache, mental confusion, loss of appetite, nervousness, chest pain or irregular heartbeat.

ANTIARRHYTHMIC

Cardioquin, Cin-Quin, Disopyramide, Duraquin, Norpace, Norpace CR, Procainamide, Procan SR, Pronestyl, Quinaglute Dura-Tabs, Quinidex Extentabs, Quinidine, Quinidine Gluconate SR, Quinora, Tonocard

THIS MEDICATION IS USED:

To make the heart beat at a normal rhythm.

PROPER USE OF THIS MEDICATION:

 Unless your doctor has told you differently, this medicine should be taken on an empty stomach with a glass of water at least 1 hour before or 2 hours after a meal to maximize absorption.

If stomach upset occurs, you may take this medicine with food unless told otherwise.

 The controlled release forms should be swallowed whole, NOT crushed or chewed.

SPECIAL INSTRUCTIONS:

 Proper control of your condition requires you to take this medicine as instructed at the same time every day, DO NOT skip a dose nor stop taking the medicine without asking your doctor.

Since this medicine does not cure but helps to control your condition, you should continue to take it even if you are feeling well.

 DO NOT take nonprescription cough/cold or diet products without asking your doctor or pharmacist.

 You may experience dizziness, blurred vision or drowsiness from this medicine. If you do, be careful driving or performing hazardous tasks.

 Alcoholic beverages can increase the drowsiness.

If you miss a dose of this medicine, take it as soon as possible. But, if it is almost time for your next dose, skip the missed dose and go back to your regular dose. DO NOT take a double dose.

DO NOT keep or use outdated medication. Keep all medication out of the reach of children.

POSSIBLE SIDE EFFECTS:

Be sure to tell your doctor if the following occur: ringing or buzzing in the ears, prolonged headache or fever, visual disturbances, persistent soreness of the mouth or throat, unusual bleeding, arthritis like symptoms, difficult breathing or cough or wheezing.

TRENTAL

THIS MEDICINE IS USED:

To improve blood flow.

PROPER USE OF THIS MEDICINE:

 This medication SHOULD be taken with food to reduce the chance of stomach upset.

 This medication should be swallowed whole, NOT crushed, broken or chewed.

SPECIAL INSTRUCTIONS:

 If stomach upset occurs and continues or becomes severe, you should contact your doctor.

It is important that you take this medicine exactly as your doctor has instructed.

If you miss a dose of this medicine, take it as soon as possible. But, if it is almost time for your next dose, skip the missed dose and go back to your regular dose. DO NOT take a double dose.

DO NOT keep or use outdated medication. Keep all medication out of the reach of children.

POSSIBLE SIDE EFFECTS:

 Be sure to tell your doctor if the following occur: nausea or vomiting, dizziness or severe headache.

BETA BLOCKER OPHTHALMIC

Betagan Ophthalmic, Betoptic Ophthalmic, Betoptic S Ophthalmic,
Ocupress Ophthalmic, Optipranolol, Timoptic Ophthalmic

THIS MEDICATION IS USED:

To treat glaucoma.

PROPER USE OF THIS MEDICATION:

Wash your hands with soap and water before using the eye drops.

Gently pull lower eyelid downward to form a pouch.

Tilt head backward, hold the dropper above the eye and drop the prescribed amount of medicine inside the lower lid.

DO NOT touch the dropper to any surface.

Release lower lid. Try not to blink for a few seconds. Replace the cap on the bottle.

The suspension forms of this medication should be shaken well just before using. If you are not sure or have not been told ask your pharmacist.

SPECIAL INSTRUCTIONS:

NEVER rinse the dropper. You may contaminate the medication.

Eye drops may blur your vision for a few minutes. If they do, DO NOT drive or perform hazardous tasks until your vision has cleared.

NEVER use eye drops that have changed color or appear to have crystals in the liquid.

Call your doctor if your condition becomes worse or if you experience itching or burning for more than a few minutes after placing drops in the eye.

If you are using more than 1 kind of eye drop at the same time, wait at least 5 minutes before you use another eye drop. Check with your doctor or pharmacist about which one to use first.

If you wear contact lenses, remove them before instilling the eye drops.

If you miss a dose of this medicine, use it as soon as possible. But, if it is almost time for your next dose, skip the missed dose and go back to your regular dose. DO NOT use a double dose.

DO NOT keep or use outdated medication. Keep all medication out of the reach of children.

In case of accidental ingestion, call your doctor or poison control center immediately.

POSSIBLE SIDE EFFECTS:

 Be sure to tell your doctor if the following occur: severe headache or dizziness, continued blurred vision or irritation, or difficulty in sleeping or breathing.

PILOCARPINE OPHTHALMIC
Isopto Carbachol Ophthalmic, Isopto Carpine Ophthalmic,
Pilagan Ophthalmic, Pilocar Ophthalmic

THIS MEDICATION IS USED:

To treat glaucoma.

PROPER USE OF THIS MEDICATION:

Wash your hands with soap and water before using the eye drops.

Gently pull lower eyelid downward to form a pouch.

Tilt head backward, hold the dropper above the eye and drop the prescribed amount of medicine inside the lower lid.

DO NOT touch the dropper to any surface.

Release lower lid. Try not to blink for a few seconds. Replace the cap on the bottle.

SPECIAL INSTRUCTIONS:

NEVER rinse the dropper. You may contaminate the medication.

Eye drops may blur your vision for a few minutes. If they do, DO NOT drive or perform hazardous tasks until your vision has cleared.

NEVER use eye drops that have changed color or appear to have crystals in the solution.

It is important that you use this medicine exactly as your doctor has instructed.

Call your doctor if your condition becomes worse or if you experience itching or burning for more than a few minutes after placing drops in the eye.

If you are using more than 1 kind of eye drop at the same time, wait at least 5 minutes before you use another eye drop. Check with your doctor or pharmacist about which one to use first.

If you wear contact lenses, remove them before instilling the eye drops.

Always keep container tightly closed when not in use.

If you miss a dose of this medicine, use it as soon as possible. But, if it is almost time for your next dose, skip the missed dose and go back to your regular dose. DO NOT use a double dose.

DO NOT keep or use outdated medication. Keep all medication out of the reach of children.

In case of accidental ingestion, call your doctor or poison control center immediately.

POSSIBLE SIDE EFFECTS:

 Be sure to tell your doctor if the following occur: severe headache, or persistent eye irritation.

BUTALBITAL/ASPIRIN
Axotal, Fiorgen PF, Fiorinal, Isollyl

THIS MEDICATION IS USED:

To treat tension headaches.

PROPER USE OF THIS MEDICATION:

 Take this medication with food and a glass of water to avoid upsetting your stomach.

SPECIAL INSTRUCTIONS:

 You may experience dizziness, blurred vision or drowsiness from this medicine. Be careful driving or performing hazardous tasks.

 Alcoholic beverages can increase drowsiness.

DO NOT change the amount of medicine taken nor stop taking it without consulting your doctor.

 Discard doses that have a strong vinegar odor. The aspirin has decomposed.

 DO NOT take nonprescription ibuprofen, aspirin or acetaminophen products while taking this drug without checking with your doctor or pharmacist.

If you miss a dose of this medicine, take it as soon as possible. But, if it is almost time for your next dose, skip the missed dose and go back to your regular dose. DO NOT take a double dose.

DO NOT keep or use outdated medication. Keep all medication out of the reach of children.

POSSIBLE SIDE EFFECTS:

 Be sure to tell your doctor if the following occur: difficulty in breathing, ringing or buzzing of the ears or reduced hearing, severe headache or stomach cramps or black tarry stools.

FIORINAL W/CODEINE

THIS MEDICATION IS USED:

To treat pain.

PROPER USE OF THIS MEDICATION:

 Take this medication with food and a glass of water to help avoid upsetting your stomach.

SPECIAL INSTRUCTIONS:

 You may experience dizziness, blurred vision or drowsiness from this medicine. If you do, be careful driving or performing hazardous tasks.

 Alcoholic beverages can increase the drowsiness.

DO NOT change the amount of medicine taken nor stop taking it without consulting your doctor.

 Discard doses that have a strong vinegar odor. The aspirin has decomposed.

 DO NOT take nonprescription ibuprofen, aspirin or acetaminophen products while taking this drug without checking with your doctor or pharmacist.

 If taken for a few days, you may experience some constipation. You should increase the amount of bulk in your diet (bran, psyllium, and fresh fruits) and drink lots of fluids.

If you miss a dose of this medicine, take it as soon as possible. But, if it is almost time for your next dose, skip the missed dose and go back to your regular dose. DO NOT take a double dose.

DO NOT keep or use outdated medication. Keep all medication out of the reach of children.

POSSIBLE SIDE EFFECTS:

 Be sure to tell your doctor if the following occur: difficulty in breathing, ringing or buzzing of the ears or reduced hearing, severe headache or stomach cramps or black tarry stools.

METRONIDAZOLE
Femazole, Flagyl, Protostat

THIS MEDICATION IS USED:

To treat infections.

PROPER USE OF THIS MEDICATION:

 Take this medicine with a glass of water. If it upsets your stomach you may take it with food.

SPECIAL INSTRUCTIONS:

There are different lengths of therapy that are considered effective. You should take all of your medicine exactly as instructed by your doctor.

 It is best to NOT drink alcoholic beverages while taking this medication and for at least one day afterward. The combination may cause headache, flushing or an upset stomach.

 This medicine may cause a darkening of your urine, DO NOT be alarmed. This is not unusual and will go away when you stop taking this medicine.

If you miss a dose, take the missed dose as soon as possible. But if it is almost time for your next dose (within 2 hours), DOUBLE that dose. Then go back to your regular dosing schedule.

DO NOT keep or use outdated medication. Keep all medication out of the reach of children.

POSSIBLE SIDE EFFECTS:

 Be sure to tell your doctor if the following occur: dizziness or lightheadedness, unusual anxiety or depression, vaginal irritation not present prior to therapy, numbness or tingling in the extremities, persistent sore throat or fever.

SELDANE

THIS MEDICATION IS USED:

To relieve the runny nose, watery eyes and sneezing of colds and hay fever. It may also be used for allergic reactions.

PROPER USE OF THIS MEDICATION:

Take this medicine with a glass of water. It may be taken with or without food.

If it upsets your stomach take it with food.

SPECIAL INSTRUCTIONS:

If your mouth becomes dry, you may suck on hard candy, chew gum or use a saliva substitute.

It is important that you take this medicine exactly as your doctor has instructed. Take this only as needed and DO NOT take more doses than prescribed by your doctor.

You should NOT take nonprescription cough/cold products without asking your doctor or pharmacist.

You should talk with your doctor before taking the following prescription medications: erythromycin derivatives, ketoconazole (Nizoral), or itraconazole (Sporanox).

Tell your doctor if you are pregnant, plan to become pregnant or are breastfeeding.

If you miss a dose of this medicine, take it as soon as possible. But, if it is almost time for your next dose, skip the missed dose and go back to your regular dosing schedule. DO NOT take a double dose.

DO NOT keep or use outdated medication. Keep all medication out of the reach of children.

POSSIBLE SIDE EFFECTS:

 Be sure to tell your doctor if the following occur: thickening of the bronchial secretions, headache, dry mouth, blurred vision, drowsiness, increased appetite, nervousness, dizziness, nausea or upset stomach, chest pain or irregular heartbeat.

AMILORIDE/HCTZ, MODURETIC

THIS MEDICATION IS USED:

To help remove excess fluid and salt, decrease swelling and treat high blood pressure.

PROPER USE OF THIS MEDICATION:

This medication should be taken with food.

SPECIAL INSTRUCTIONS:

This medicine may cause lightheadedness. Sit or lie down at the first signs. Avoid sudden changes in posture. Be careful going up and down stairs.

Proper control of your condition requires you to take this medicine as instructed at the same time every day, DO NOT skip a dose nor stop taking the medicine without asking your doctor.

Since this medicine does not cure but helps to control your condition, you should continue to take it even if you are feeling well.

You should NOT use salt substitutes without asking your doctor or pharmacist.

DO NOT take nonprescription cough/cold or diet products without asking your doctor or pharmacist.

This medicine may make your skin more sensitive to sunlight or sunlamps. Ask your pharmacist about a suitable sunblock product (of at least SPF 15) to minimize problems during exposure.

If you miss a dose of this medicine, take it as soon as possible. But, if it is almost time for your next dose, skip the missed dose and go back to your regular dose. DO NOT take a double dose.

DO NOT keep or use outdated medication. Keep all medication out of the reach of children.

POSSIBLE SIDE EFFECTS:

 Be sure to tell your doctor if the following occur: light-headedness, nausea or vomiting or muscle weakness or cramps, sore throat or yellow coloration of the eyes or skin.

MAXZIDE
Triamterene w/Hydrochlorothiazide

THIS MEDICATION IS USED:

To help remove excess fluid and salt, decrease swelling and treat high blood pressure.

PROPER USE OF THIS MEDICATION:

You should take this medicine at the same time every day. The best time is in the morning before breakfast. If stomach upset occurs, you may take this medication with food unless told otherwise.

SPECIAL INSTRUCTIONS:

This medicine may cause lightheadedness. Sit or lie down at the first signs. Avoid sudden changes in posture. Be careful going up and down stairs.

Proper control of your condition requires you to take this medicine as instructed at the same time every day, DO NOT skip a dose nor stop taking the medicine without asking your doctor.

Since this medicine does not cure but helps to control your condition, you should continue to take it even if you are feeling well.

You should NOT use salt substitutes without asking your doctor or pharmacist.

DO NOT take nonprescription cough/cold or diet products without asking your doctor or pharmacist.

This medicine may make your skin more sensitive to sunlight or sunlamps. Ask your pharmacist about a suitable sunblock product (of at least SPF 15) to minimize problems during exposure.

If you miss a dose of this medicine, take it as soon as possible. But, if it is almost time for your next dose, skip the missed dose and go back to your regular dose. DO NOT take a double dose.

DO NOT keep or use outdated medication. Keep all medication out of the reach of children.

POSSIBLE SIDE EFFECTS:

 Be sure to tell your doctor if the following occur: lightheadedness, nausea or vomiting or muscle weakness or cramps, sore throat or yellow coloration of the eyes or skin.

CATAPRES TTS

THIS MEDICATION IS USED:

 To treat high blood pressure.

PROPER USE OF THIS MEDICATION:

 Apply the patch as directed by your doctor or pharmacist (usually once every 7 days) to a skin area free of hair on the upper arm or body.

 Rotate application sites to avoid irritation.

The patch can be worn when you bathe or shower.

If the patch falls off, replace it and hold it on with the adhesive bandage supplied in the box.

Use a different area on the skin each time you apply the patch. REMOVE THE OLD PATCH.

SPECIAL INSTRUCTIONS:

 This medicine may cause you to be drowsy the first few days you use it or when your doctor increases the amount you are using. If it does, be careful driving or performing hazardous tasks.

 This medicine may cause lightheadedness. Sit or lie down at the first signs. Avoid sudden changes in posture. Be careful going up and down stairs.

Alcoholic beverages can increase the drowsiness.

 Proper control of your condition requires you to use this medicine as instructed at the same time every day, DO NOT skip a dose nor stop using the medicine without asking your doctor.

Since this medicine does not cure but helps to control your condition, you should continue to use it even if you are feeling well.

DO NOT take nonprescription cough/cold or diet products without asking your doctor or pharmacist.

If you miss a dose of this medicine, use it as soon as possible. But, if it is missed for 3 or more days, check with your doctor.

DO NOT keep or use outdated medication. Keep all medication out of the reach of children.

POSSIBLE SIDE EFFECTS:

 Be sure to tell your doctor if the following occur: chest pain, unusual swelling, weakness, constipation, dry mouth or excessive tiredness.

LITHIUM
Eskalith, Eskalith-CR, Lithane, Lithium Carbonate, Lithobid

THIS MEDICATION IS USED:
To treat manic-depressive illness.

PROPER USE OF THIS MEDICATION:

 Take this medicine with a glass of water. If it upsets your stomach you may take it with food.

 The controlled release forms should be swallowed whole, NOT crushed or chewed.

If you are taking the liquid form, it should be diluted in water or juice just before taking.

SPECIAL INSTRUCTIONS:

 You may experience dizziness, blurred vision or drowsiness from this medicine. If you do, be careful driving or performing hazardous tasks.

Alcoholic beverages can increase the drowsiness.

 This medicine may cause lightheadedness. Sit or lie down at the first signs. Avoid sudden changes in posture. Be careful going up and down stairs.

 Proper control of your condition requires you to take this medicine as instructed at the same time every day, DO NOT skip a dose nor stop taking the medicine without asking your doctor.

Since this medicine does not cure but helps to control your condition, you should continue to take it even if you are feeling well.

 It is recommended that you drink lots of fluids and NOT increase your salt intake and NOT use salt substitutes while taking this medicine without asking your doctor or pharmacist.

If you miss a dose of this medicine, take it as soon as possible. But, if it is almost time for your next dose, skip the missed dose and go back to your regular dose. DO NOT take a double dose.

DO NOT keep or use outdated medication. Keep all medication out of the reach of children.

POSSIBLE SIDE EFFECTS:

Be sure to tell your doctor if the following occur: vomiting, diarrhea, excessive thirst, urination or drowsiness, tremors, confusion, unusual weight gain or lack of coordination.

ESTROGENS
Estinyl, Estrovis, Feminone, Menest, Ogen, Premarin

THIS MEDICATION IS USED:

For several different medical reasons, such as, alleviating the symptoms of menopause and treating osteoporosis (loss of bone mass).

PROPER USE OF THIS MEDICATION:

 Take this medicine with a glass of water. If it upsets your stomach you may take it with food.

SPECIAL INSTRUCTIONS:

 A detailed leaflet is available with your prescription. Read it and follow its instructions. If you have any questions or need help understanding it, ask your doctor or pharmacist.

 If there is a chance that pregnancy has occurred stop taking this medication and call your doctor right away.

If you miss a dose of this medicine, take it as soon as possible. But, if it is almost time for your next dose, skip the missed dose and go back to your regular dose. DO NOT take a double dose.

DO NOT keep or use outdated medication. Keep all medication out of the reach of children.

POSSIBLE SIDE EFFECTS:

 Be sure to tell your doctor if the following occur: stomach cramps, loss of appetite, nausea, breast tenderness, swelling of the extremities, yellow coloration of the skin or eyes, abnormal vaginal bleeding, pains in the calves or chest or difficult breathing, severe headache or blurred vision.

DOLOBID, DIFLUNISAL

THIS MEDICATION IS USED:

For the relief of pain. It can also be used to relieve swelling in certain kinds of arthritis.

PROPER USE OF THIS MEDICATION:

 This medication should be taken with a glass of water. If stomach upset occurs, you may take it with food or milk.

 This medication should be swallowed whole, NOT crushed or chewed.

SPECIAL INSTRUCTIONS:

If this medicine is used for arthritis, it must be taken regularly as ordered by your doctor.

 DO NOT take nonprescription ibuprofen, aspirin or acetaminophen products while taking this drug without checking with your doctor or pharmacist.

 You may experience dizziness, blurred vision or drowsiness from this medicine. If you do, be careful driving or performing hazardous tasks.

If you miss a dose of this medicine, take it as soon as possible. But, if it is almost time for your next dose, skip the missed dose and take your regular dose. DO NOT take a double dose.

DO NOT keep or use outdated medication. Keep all medication out of the reach of children.

POSSIBLE SIDE EFFECTS:

 Be sure to tell your doctor if any of the following occur: skin rash, ringing or buzzing in the ears, changed vision, stomach pain or nausea, persistent sore throat or fever, black, tarry or bloody stools, unusual weight gain or edema in the extremities or difficulty in breathing.

CYCLOBENZAPRINE, FLEXERIL

THIS MEDICATION IS USED:

For short term (2-3 weeks) use to relax muscles and to relieve muscle pain and discomfort.

PROPER USE OF THIS MEDICATION:

 Take this medicine with a glass of water. If it upsets your stomach you may take it with food.

SPECIAL INSTRUCTIONS:

 You may experience dizziness, blurred vision or drowsiness from this medicine. If you do, be careful driving or performing hazardous tasks.

Alcoholic beverages can increase the drowsiness.

 This medicine may cause lightheadedness. Sit or lie down at the first signs. Avoid sudden changes in posture. Be careful going up and down stairs.

DO NOT change the amount of medicine taken nor stop taking it without consulting your doctor.

 DO NOT take nonprescription cough/cold, hay fever, diet or sleep aid products without asking your doctor or pharmacist.

 If taken for a few days, you may experience some constipation. You should increase the amount of bulk in your diet (bran, psyllium, and fresh fruits) and drink lots of fluids.

 This medicine may make your skin more sensitive to sunlight or sunlamps. Ask your pharmacist about a suitable sunblock product (of at least SPF 15) to minimize problems during exposure.

If you miss a dose of this medicine, take it as soon as possible. But, if it is almost time for your next dose, skip the

missed dose and go back to your regular dose. DO NOT take a double dose.

DO NOT keep or use outdated medication. Keep all medication out of the reach of children.

POSSIBLE SIDE EFFECTS:

 Be sure to tell your doctor if the following occur: blurred vision or eye pain, nervousness or confusion, irregular heartbeat or pulse, fainting spells, difficulty sleeping or urinating, severe drowsiness, troubled breathing or hallucinations.

AUGMENTIN

THIS MEDICATION IS USED:

To treat infections.

PROPER USE OF THIS MEDICATION:

 This medication should be taken with a glass of water and it can be taken with or without food.

 If you are taking the liquid form, it should be stored in the refrigerator and used within 10 days. The contents should be shaken well just before measuring the dose. There are special measuring devices available, ask your pharmacist for one.

 If you are taking the chewable form, it should be chewed well before swallowing.

SPECIAL INSTRUCTIONS:

 The recommended length of treatment is 7-10 days. You should take all the medication unless otherwise instructed by your doctor.

 If you experience diarrhea while taking this medicine, DO NOT take any antidiarrheal medicine without first asking your doctor or pharmacist.

If you miss a dose, take the missed dose as soon as possible. But if it is almost time for your next dose (within 2 hours), DOUBLE that dose. Then go back to your regular dosing schedule.

DO NOT keep or use outdated medication. Keep all medication out of the reach of children.

POSSIBLE SIDE EFFECTS:

 Be sure to tell your doctor if the following occur: skin rash, hives or itching, shortness of breath or wheezing, swelling of the face, prolonged nausea, vomiting or diarrhea, black tongue, or persistent sore throat or fever.

MECLIZINE, ANTIVERT

THIS MEDICATION IS USED:

To treat nausea, vomiting and dizziness associated with motion sickness. It is also used to treat certain types of vertigo.

PROPER USE OF THIS MEDICATION:

 Take this medicine with a glass of water. If it upsets your stomach you may take it with food.

 If you are taking the chewable form, it should be chewed well before swallowing.

If you are taking this medicine to prevent motion sickness, take it about 1 hour before you begin to travel.

SPECIAL INSTRUCTIONS:

 You may experience dizziness, blurred vision or drowsiness from this medicine. If you do, be careful driving or performing hazardous tasks.

 Alcoholic beverages can increase the drowsiness.

If your mouth becomes dry, you may suck on hard candy, chew gum or use a saliva substitute.

 You should NOT take nonprescription cough and cold products without first checking with your doctor or pharmacist.

If you miss a dose of this medicine, take it as soon as possible. But, if it is almost time for your next dose, skip the missed dose and go back to your regular dosing schedule. DO NOT take a double dose.

DO NOT keep or use outdated medication. Keep all medication out of the reach of children.

POSSIBLE SIDE EFFECTS:

 Be sure to tell your doctor if the following occur: drowsiness, blurred vision, dryness of the mouth, nose or throat and loss of appetite.

HYDERGINE
Ergoloid Mesylates, Ergoloid Mesylates Sublingual,
Hydergine LC, Hydergine Sublingual

THIS MEDICINE IS USED:

To treat changes in mood, memory or behavior, due to the
aging process or some underlying dementing condition
(Alzheimer's or senility).

PROPER USE OF THIS MEDICINE:

 Take this medicine with a glass of water. If it upsets your
stomach you may take it with food.

 If you are using the sublingual form, dissolve the tablet
under the tongue. DO NOT chew or swallow it whole.

DO NOT eat, drink or smoke while this medicine is dissolving in your mouth.

 If you are taking the liquid form, measure the dose using
the specially designed measuring device provided with your
medication. If you have any questions concerning how to
measure your dose, ask your pharmacist.

The medicine can be diluted in water or juice.

SPECIAL INSTRUCTIONS:

 It may take several weeks before the full effects of this
medicine are noticed. DO NOT change the amount of
medicine taken nor stop taking it without consulting
your doctor.

If you miss a dose of this medicine, take it as soon as possible. But, if it is almost time for your next dose, skip the
missed dose and go back to your regular dose. DO NOT
take a double dose.

DO NOT keep or use outdated medication. Keep all medication out of the reach of children.

In case of accidental overdose contact your poison control
center immediately.

POSSIBLE SIDE EFFECTS:

 Be sure to tell your doctor if the following occur: prolonged nausea, or sores in the mouth or on the tongue.

CARBAMAZEPINE, TEGRETOL

THIS MEDICATION IS USED:

To control convulsions and seizures.

PROPER USE OF THIS MEDICATION:

 To maximize absorption and reduce the chance of stomach upset, take this medicine with food.

 If you are taking the liquid form, the contents should be shaken vigorously just before measuring the dose. There are special measuring devices available, ask your pharmacist if you want one.

 If you are taking the chewable form, it should be chewed well before swallowing.

SPECIAL INSTRUCTIONS:

 You may experience dizziness, blurred vision or drowsiness from this medicine. If you do, be careful driving or performing hazardous tasks.

Alcoholic beverages can increase the drowsiness.

 Proper control of your condition requires you to take this medicine as instructed at the same time every day, DO NOT skip a dose nor stop taking the medicine without asking your doctor.

 This medicine may make your skin more sensitive to sunlight or sunlamps. Ask your pharmacist about a suitable sunblock product (of at least SPF 15) to minimize problems during exposure.

If you miss a dose of this medicine, take it as soon as possible. But, if it is almost time for your next dose, skip the missed dose and go back to your regular dose. DO NOT take a double dose.

DO NOT keep or use outdated medication. Keep all medication out of the reach of children.

POSSIBLE SIDE EFFECTS:

Be sure to tell your doctor if the following occur: eye pain, confusion, irregular heartbeat or pulse, fainting spells or difficult breathing.

MUSCLE RELAXANT

Carisoprodol, Chlorzoxazone, Marbaxin, Metaxalone,
Methocarbamol, Norflex, Orphenadrine, Paraflex, Parafon
Forte DSC, Rela, Robaxin, Robomol, Skelaxin, Soma, Soprodol

THIS MEDICATION IS USED:

To relax muscles and to relieve muscle pain and discomfort.

PROPER USE OF THIS MEDICATION:

 Take this medicine with a glass of water. If it upsets your stomach you may take it with food.

SPECIAL INSTRUCTIONS:

 You may experience dizziness, blurred vision or drowsiness from this medicine. Be careful driving or performing hazardous tasks.

Alcoholic beverages can increase the drowsiness.

 This medicine may cause lightheadedness. Sit or lie down at the first signs. Avoid sudden changes in posture. Be careful going up and down stairs.

DO NOT change the amount of medicine taken nor stop taking it without consulting your doctor.

 If taken for a few days, you may experience some constipation. You should increase the amount of bulk in your diet (bran, psyllium, and fresh fruits) and drink lots of fluids.

If you miss a dose of this medicine, take it as soon as possible. But, if it is almost time for your next dose, skip the missed dose and go back to your regular dose. DO NOT take a double dose.

DO NOT keep or use outdated medication. Keep all medication out of the reach of children.

POSSIBLE SIDE EFFECTS:

 Be sure to tell your doctor if the following occur: nausea and vomiting, troubled breathing, skin rash, blurred vision, severe headache, persistent sore throat or fever, irregular heartbeat or yellow coloration of the skin.

CIPRO

THIS MEDICATION IS USED:

To treat infections.

PROPER USE OF THIS MEDICATION:

 This medication can be taken with or without food. The best time is two hours after a meal, followed by a glass of water.

If stomach upsets occurs, take it with food.

DO NOT take antacids or iron supplements within 2 hours of taking this medication.

SPECIAL INSTRUCTIONS:

 The recommended length of treatment is 7-10 days. You should take all the medication unless otherwise instructed by your doctor.

 It is recommended that you drink lots of fluids while you are taking this medication.

 You may experience dizziness, blurred vision or drowsiness from this medicine. If you do, be careful driving or performing hazardous tasks.

 This medicine may make your skin more sensitive to sunlight or sunlamps. Ask your pharmacist about a suitable sunblock product (of at least SPF 15) to minimize problems during exposure.

Stop this medicine at the first sign of a skin rash or other allergic reaction and tell your doctor.

Be careful taking products containing caffeine while on this medicine, as there may be increased caffeine-related stimulation.

If you miss a dose of this medicine, take it as soon as possible. But, if it is almost time for your next dose, skip the missed dose and go back to your regular dosing schedule.

DO NOT take a double dose.

DO NOT keep or use outdated medication. Keep all medication out of the reach of children.

POSSIBLE SIDE EFFECTS:

 Be sure to tell your doctor if the following occur: skin rash, nausea or vomiting, headache, diarrhea, blurred vision, dizziness or drowsiness, stomach pain or dry mouth.

NITROFURANTOIN
Furadantin, Macrobid, Macrodantin

THIS MEDICATION IS USED:

To treat infections.

PROPER USE OF THIS MEDICATION:

 To maximize absorption and to reduce the chance of stomach upset, this medicine SHOULD be taken with food.

 The liquid form of this medication should be shaken well just before measuring the dose. There are special measuring devices available, ask your pharmacist if you want one.

SPECIAL INSTRUCTION:

 For most urinary tract infections the recommended length of treatment is for at least one week and should continue for at least 3 days after the infection is eradicated. You should take all the medication unless otherwise instructed by your doctor.

 This medicine may cause a darkening of your urine, DO NOT be alarmed. This is not unusual and will go away when you stop taking the medicine.

If you miss a dose, take the missed dose as soon as possible. But if it is almost time for your next dose (within 2 hours), DOUBLE that dose Then go back to your regular dosing schedule.

DO NOT keep or use outdated medication. Keep all medication out of the reach of children.

POSSIBLE SIDE EFFECTS:

 Be sure to tell your doctor if the following occur: chest pain. cough, difficult breathing, chills or fever, dizziness or drowsiness, headache, numbness or tingling in the extremities.

TRIAVIL/ETRAFON
Perphenazine/Amitriptyline

THIS MEDICATION IS USED:

To treat emotional problems that are characterized by intermittent periods of anxiety, agitation and depression.

PROPER USE OF THIS MEDICATION:

Take this medicine with a glass of water. If it upsets your stomach you may take it with food.

DO NOT take within 1-2 hours of an antacid.

SPECIAL INSTRUCTIONS:

You may experience dizziness, blurred vision or drowsiness from this medicine. If you do, be careful driving or performing hazardous tasks.

Alcoholic beverages can increase the drowsiness.

This medicine may cause lightheadedness. Sit or lie down at the first signs. Avoid sudden changes in posture. Be careful going up and down stairs.

DO NOT take nonprescription cough/cold, hay fever, antacids, antidiarrheals, diet or sleep aid products without asking your doctor or pharmacist.

If your mouth becomes dry, you may suck on hard candy, chew gum or use a saliva substitute.

If taken for a few days, you may experience some constipation. You should increase the amount of bulk in your diet (bran, psyllium, and fresh fruits) and drink lots of fluids.

This medicine may make your skin more sensitive to sunlight or sunlamps. Ask your pharmacist about a suitable sunblock product (of at least SPF 15) to minimize problems during exposure.

If you miss a dose of this medicine, take it as soon as possible. But, if it is almost time for your next dose, skip the missed dose and go back to your regular dose. DO NOT take a double dose.

DO NOT keep or use outdated medication. Keep all medication out of the reach of children.

POSSIBLE SIDE EFFECTS:

 Be sure to tell your doctor if the following occur: blurred vision or eye pain, nervousness or confusion, irregular heartbeat or pulse, fainting spells, difficulty getting to sleep or urinating, severe drowsiness, troubled breathing, high fever or hallucinations or yellow coloring of the skin.

APPETITE SUPPRESSANT

Adipex-P, Bontril Pdm, Bontril SR, Didrex, Diethylpropion,
Fastin, Ionamin, Mazanor, Mazindol, Phendimetrazine,
Phentermine, Plegine, Pondimin, Prelu-2, Sanorex,
Tenuate, Tenuate Dospan, Tepanil, Tepanil Ten-Tab

THIS MEDICATION IS USED:

For the treatment of obesity as a short term adjunct in a
regimen of weight control based on caloric restriction.

PROPER USE OF THIS MEDICATION:

 This medicine should only be taken a few weeks (8-12
weeks) in combination with a diet and exercise plan that
will help lose weight.

 Some products should be taken once daily in the morning.
Others, should be taken 2-3 times a day one hour before
meals. The once daily dose forms of this medication should
be swallowed whole, DO NOT crush or chew. If you have
any questions about how to take your medication check
with your doctor or pharmacist.

SPECIAL INSTRUCTIONS:

 When taken too late in the day, this medicine may cause
trouble in getting to sleep. If you are having problems
sleeping contact your doctor.

 While this medication does not directly cause drowsiness,
it may mask fatigue until the point that drowsiness occurs.
Therefore you should be careful driving or performing hazardous tasks.

 DO NOT take nonprescription cough/cold or diet products without asking your doctor or pharmacist.

If you miss a dose of this medicine, take it as soon as possible. But, if it is almost time for your next dose, skip the
missed dose and go back to your regular dose. DO NOT
take a double dose.

DO NOT keep or use outdated medication. Keep all medication out of the reach of children.

POSSIBLE SIDE EFFECTS:

 Be sure to tell your doctor if the following occur: irregular heartbeat, or chest pain, changes in mood or severe headache.

INSULIN
Humulin, Iletin, Mixtard, Mixtard Human, Novolin

THIS MEDICATION IS USED:
To treat diabetes.

PROPER USE OF THIS MEDICATION:

PREPARING YOUR DOSE OF INSULIN

Wash your hands.

Gently roll the insulin bottle in your hands several times to mix the insulin. DO NOT SHAKE the bottle. Flip off the cap, but DO NOT remove the rubber stopper.

Wipe the top of the bottle with an alcohol swab.

Remove the needle cover from the syringe. Draw air into the syringe by pulling back on the plunger. The amount of air should be equal to your insulin dose.

Insert the needle through the rubber top of the insulin bottle. Push the plunger in. The air that was injected into the bottle will allow the insulin to be easily withdrawn.

Turn the bottle and syringe upside down in one hand. With your hand, draw back on the plunger slowly to obtain the correct dose.

Check the syringe for air bubbles. To remove air bubbles, push the air bubbles slowly back into the bottle by pressing on the needle plunger. Then measure the correct dose of insulin.

Double-check your dose.

Remove the needle from bottle. Cover the needle carefully with the needle cap.

INJECTING YOUR DOSE OF INSULIN

Cleanse the skin where the injection is to be made (on thighs, buttocks, abdomen, or upper arms) with an alcohol swab and let the area dry.

With one hand, stabilize the skin by pinching it up and holding it firmly. Pick up the syringe with the other hand and insert the needle into the skin (90 degree angle).

To inject the insulin, push the plunger all the way down, using less than five (5) seconds to inject the dose.

Hold an alcohol swab near the needle and pull it straight out of the skin. Press the alcohol swab over the injection site for several seconds. DO NOT rub. Dispose of syringe in a proper container.

If you are taking more than one (1) injection of insulin per day, use a new syringe every time unless otherwise directed by your doctor, nurse or pharmacist. Repeat above procedures.

SPECIAL INSTRUCTIONS:

When buying insulin, always check the expiration date to make sure the insulin will be used before it expires.

DO NOT change the strength or type of insulin unless told to do so by your doctor.

Your pharmacist can advise you on the various types of diabetic testing products on the market and their proper procedures for use.

 DO NOT take nonprescription cough/cold, aspirin or diet products without asking your doctor or pharmacist.

 DO NOT drink alcoholic beverages before checking with your doctor.

 Call your doctor if you develop any signs of hyperglycemia (high blood sugar) or hypoglycemia (low blood sugar).

SIGNS OF HYPERGLYCEMIA – HIGH BLOOD SUGAR:

Excessive thirst and or urination, dry mouth, drowsiness, flushed dry skin, fruit-like breath odor, stomach ache, nausea or vomiting, difficult breathing. This can be caused by a missed insulin dose, overeating, not following your diet, or if you have a fever or an infection.

SIGNS OF HYPOGLYCEMIA – LOW BLOOD SUGAR:

Anxiety, chills, cold sweats, cool pale skin, confusion, drowsiness, excessive hunger, unusual tiredness or weakness. This can be caused by too much insulin, missing a snack or meal, sickness, too much exercise, drinking alcohol or taking certain medications. If these symptoms occur, you should eat or drink a product containing sugar such as orange juice, corn syrup, honey, sugar cubes or table sugar.

DO NOT keep or use outdated medication. Keep all medication out of the reach of children.

LOPID, GEMFIBROZIL

THIS MEDICATION IS USED:

To lower cholesterol and triglyceride levels in the blood.

PROPER USE OF THIS MEDICATION:

 Take this medicine 30 minutes before the morning and evening meals.

SPECIAL INSTRUCTIONS:

 You should follow a standard cholesterol lowering diet while taking this medicine. Your diet is the MOST important part of controlling your condition and is necessary if the medicine is to work properly.

 Proper control of your condition requires you to take this medicine as instructed at the same time every day, DO NOT skip a dose nor stop taking the medicine without asking your doctor.

If you miss a dose of this medicine, take it as soon as possible. But, if it is almost time for your next dose, skip the missed dose and go back to your regular dose. DO NOT take a double dose.

DO NOT keep or use outdated medication. Keep all medication out of the reach of children.

POSSIBLE SIDE EFFECTS:

 Be sure to tell your doctor if the following occur: stomach upset, diarrhea, nausea or vomiting, dizziness, blurred vision or headache, muscle pain or weakness.

MEVACOR

THIS MEDICATION IS USED:

To lower levels of cholesterol in the blood.

PROPER USE OF THIS MEDICATION:

 Take this medicine with food to maximize absorption (the evening meal is the best time).

SPECIAL INSTRUCTIONS:

 You should follow a standard cholesterol lowering diet while taking this medicine. Your diet is the MOST important part of controlling your condition and is necessary if the medicine is to work properly.

DO NOT stop or change the amount of medicine taken without first consulting your doctor.

If you miss a dose of this medicine, take it as soon as possible. But, if it is almost time for your next dose, skip the missed dose and go back to your regular dosing schedule. DO NOT take a double dose.

DO NOT keep or use outdated medication. Keep all medication out of the reach of children.

POSSIBLE SIDE EFFECTS:

 Be sure to tell your doctor if the following occur: blurred vision, muscle pain, tenderness or weakness, tiredness, fever, stomach pain, headache, nausea or skin rash.

CHOLESTYRAMINE POWDER
Colestid, Questran

THIS MEDICATION IS USED:

For a number of conditions, including lowering high cholesterol levels in the blood and removing high levels of bile acids due to liver problems.

PROPER USE OF THIS MEDICATION:

DO NOT take this medicine in its dry form.

MIX the powder with 4 to 6 ounces of water or noncarbonated liquid.

The mixture should be stirred to a uniform consistency and then swallowed. You may rinse the glass with more liquid to get all the medicine.

As an alternative, this medicine can be mixed with highly fluid soups or pulpy fruits with high moisture content such as applesauce, cranberry sauce or crushed pineapple.

SPECIAL INSTRUCTIONS:

You should follow a standard cholesterol lowering diet while taking this medicine. Your diet is the MOST important part of controlling your condition and is necessary if the medicine is to work properly.

Proper control of your condition requires you to take this medicine as instructed at the same time every day, DO NOT skip a dose nor stop taking the medicine without asking your doctor.

This medicine may change the effect of other medicines you are taking. It should be taken 1 hour after or 4 hours before other medications.

It is recommended that you drink lots of fluids while taking this medication.

If you miss a dose of this medicine, take it as soon as possible. But, if it is almost time for your next dose, skip the missed dose and go back to your regular dose. DO NOT take a double dose.

DO NOT keep or use outdated medication. Keep all medication out of the reach of children.

POSSIBLE SIDE EFFECTS:

 Be sure to tell your doctor if the following occur: constipation, nausea or stomach discomfort.

MONOAMINE OXIDASE INHIBITOR
Marplan, Nardil, Parnate

THIS MEDICATION IS USED:

To relieve depression.

PROPER USE OF THIS MEDICATION:

 Take this medicine with a glass of water. If it upsets your stomach you may take it with food.

SPECIAL INSTRUCTIONS:

 This medicine may cause lightheadedness. Sit or lie down at the first signs. Avoid sudden changes in posture. Be careful going up and down stairs. Avoid prolonged standing.

 You may experience dizziness, blurred vision or drowsiness from this medicine. If you do, be careful driving or performing hazardous tasks.

Alcoholic beverages can increase the drowsiness.

 DO NOT take nonprescription cough/cold or diet products without asking your doctor or pharmacist.

It may take several weeks before the full effects of this medicine are noticed. DO NOT change the amount of medicine taken nor stop taking it without consulting your doctor.

 Certain foods (those high in a substance called tyramine), beverages or other medicines taken with this medicine may cause a very dangerous reaction, SUDDEN AND EXCESSIVE RISE IN BLOOD PRESSURE. The following is a suggested list of foods and beverages to avoid: aged cheeses, (in general, avoid foods in which aging is used to increase the flavor), wines, (especially Chianti) and beer, chicken livers, fermented sausages (i.e. salami, pepperoni, summer sausage), broad beans, bananas, meats prepared with tenderizers, soy sauce, chocolate, avocados, and excessive amounts of caffeine (coffee, tea or colas). If you want a more complete list or if you have any questions, ask your doctor or pharmacist.

The effects of this medication, including its reactions with food and other medications, may last for up to two weeks after discontinuing it.

If you miss a dose of this medicine, take it as soon as possible. But, if it is almost time for your next dose, skip the missed dose and go back to your regular dose. DO NOT take a double dose.

DO NOT keep or use outdated medication. Keep all medication out of the reach of children.

POSSIBLE SIDE EFFECTS:

 Be sure to tell your doctor if the following occur: chest pain, severe headache, nausea or vomiting, stiff neck, rapid heartbeat, swelling in the extremities, yellowing of the skin.

ORAL CONTRACEPTIVE

Brevicon, Demulen, Enovid, Genora, Jenest, Levlen, Lo/Ovral, Loestrin, Loestrin-FE, Modicon, Nelova, Nordette, Norethin, Norinyl, Norlestrin, Ortho Novum, Ortho Tri-Cyclen, Ortho-Cyclen, Ovcon, Ovral, Ovrette, Tri-Levlen, Tri-Norinyl, Triphasil

THIS MEDICATION IS USED:

To prevent pregnancy and to treat various hormonal and menstrual disorders.

PROPER USE OF THIS MEDICATION:

Take this medicine at the same time every day. For this medicine to work properly, there has to be a constant level in your body. To help keep the amount constant, DO NOT miss any doses.

It is best to take this medication with the evening meal or at bedtime.

SPECIAL INSTRUCTIONS:

A detailed leaflet is available with your prescription. Read it and follow its instructions. If you have any questions or need help understanding it, ask your doctor or pharmacist.

If there is a chance that pregnancy has occurred stop taking this medication and call your doctor right away.

You should see your doctor at least once every 6-12 months for follow-up examinations while you are taking this medicine.

Some other medications may alter the effectiveness of your birth control pills. Tell all your doctors that you are taking birth control pills.

It is recommended that you NOT smoke while you are taking this medicine. Smoking while taking this medicine may increase your risk of heart disease.

MISSED DOSES:

If you miss one daily dose, take the tablet as soon as you remember and continue your regular schedule.

If you miss two daily doses in a row, take 2 tablets daily for the next 2 days, then resume your regular schedule. Report this to your doctor. You may want to use some additional form of birth control for at least the next seven days to avoid pregnancy.

If you miss three or more daily doses or more in a row, stop taking the medicine and contact your doctor. Depending on the time of month, conception is likely to occur when more than two days of birth control pills are missed.

Your doctor may think it is best to rule out the chance of pregnancy before you start taking this medicine again.

DO NOT keep or use outdated medication. Keep all medication out of the reach of children.

POSSIBLE SIDE EFFECTS:

Be sure to tell your doctor if the following occur: stomach cramps, loss of appetite, nausea, breast tenderness, swelling of the extremities, yellow coloration of the skin, abnormal vaginal bleeding, pains in the calves or chest, difficult breathing, severe headache or blurred vision.

MEXITIL

THIS MEDICATION IS USED:

To make the heart beat at a normal rhythm.

PROPER USE OF THIS MEDICATION:

 This medication SHOULD be taken with food or with an antacid to reduce stomach upset.

SPECIAL INSTRUCTIONS:

 Proper control of your condition requires you to take this medicine as instructed at the same time every day, DO NOT skip a dose nor stop taking the medicine without asking your doctor.

Since this medicine does not cure but helps to control your condition, you should continue to take it even if you are feeling well.

 DO NOT take nonprescription cough/cold or diet products without asking your doctor or pharmacist.

 You may experience dizziness, blurred vision or drowsiness from this medicine. If you do, be careful driving or performing hazardous tasks.

 Alcoholic beverages can increase the drowsiness.

If you miss a dose of this medicine, take it as soon as possible. But, if it is almost time for your next dose, skip the missed dose and go back to your regular dose. DO NOT take a double dose.

DO NOT keep or use outdated medication. Keep all medication out of the reach of children.

POSSIBLE SIDE EFFECTS:

 Be sure to tell your doctor if the following occur: ringing or buzzing in the ears, prolonged headache or fever, visual disturbances, persistent soreness of the mouth or throat, unusual bleeding, arthritis like symptoms, difficult breathing or cough or wheezing.

DECONGESTANT & EXPECTORANT

Ami-Tex, Ami-Tex LA, Banex, Deconsal II, Deconsal LA, Deconsal Sprinkle, Endal Tablet, Entex, Entex LA, Entex PSE, Guaifed, Guaifed-PD, Guiatex PSE, Histalet X, Nolex LA, Phenylpropanolamine w/Guiafenesin, Rutuss DE, Tuss LA, Vanex LA, Zephrex, Zephrex LA

THIS MEDICATION IS USED:

To relieve the symptoms of nasal stuffiness, due to colds, hay fever and allergies.

PROPER USE OF THIS MEDICATION:

 Take this medicine with a glass of water. If it upsets your stomach you may take it with food.

If you are taking the liquid form, the contents may be measured in specially designed measuring devices, ask your pharmacist if you want one.

 The pellet and controlled release forms should be swallowed whole, NOT crushed or chewed.

SPECIAL INSTRUCTIONS:

 DO NOT take nonprescription cough/cold or diet products without asking your doctor or pharmacist.

 It is recommended that you drink lots of fluids while taking this medication.

If you miss a dose of this medicine, take it as soon as possible. But, if it is almost time for your next dose, skip the missed dose and go back to your regular dose. DO NOT take a double dose.

DO NOT keep or use outdated medication. Keep all medication out of the reach of children.

POSSIBLE SIDE EFFECTS:

 Be sure to tell your doctor if the following occur: persistent headache, restlessness, prolonged nausea, or difficulty in sleeping or urination.

ANTIHYPERTENSIVE, ALPHA BLOCKER
Cardura, Hytrin, Minipress, Prazosin

THIS MEDICATION IS USED:

To treat high blood pressure.

PROPER USE OF THIS MEDICATION:

This medication should be taken with a glass of water and it can be taken with or without food.

If stomach upset occurs, you may take this medicine with food.

SPECIAL INSTRUCTIONS:

This medicine may cause you to be drowsy the first few days you take it or when your doctor increases the amount you are taking. If it does, be careful driving or performing hazardous tasks.

Alcoholic beverages can increase drowsiness while taking this medicine.

This medicine may cause lightheadedness. Sit or lie down at the first signs. Avoid sudden changes in posture. Be careful going up and down stairs.

Proper control of your condition requires you to take this medicine as instructed at the same time every day, DO NOT skip a dose nor stop taking the medicine without asking your doctor.

Since this medicine does not cure but helps to control your condition, you should continue to take it even if you are feeling well.

DO NOT take nonprescription cough/cold or diet products without asking your doctor or pharmacist.

If you miss a dose of this medicine, take it as soon as possible. But, if it is almost time for your next dose, skip the

missed dose and go back to your regular dose. DO NOT take a double dose.

DO NOT keep or use outdated medication. Keep all medication out of the reach of children.

POSSIBLE SIDE EFFECTS:

 Be sure to tell your doctor if the following occur: drowsiness, headache, skin rash, nausea, lightheadedness, fainting, chest pain, unusual swelling or weight gain.

PROGESTIN
Amen, Medroxyprogesterone, Provera

THIS MEDICATION IS USED:

For several different menstrual and hormonal problems.

PROPER USE OF THIS MEDICATION:

 Take this medicine with a glass of water. If it upsets your stomach you may take it with food.

SPECIAL INSTRUCTIONS:

 A detailed leaflet is available with your prescription. Read it and follow its instructions. If you have any questions or need help understanding it, ask your doctor or pharmacist.

 If there is a chance that pregnancy has occurred stop taking this medication and call your doctor right away.

If vaginal bleeding occurs or persists for an unusually long period, while you are taking this medication, check with your doctor.

If you miss a dose of this medicine, take it as soon as possible. But, if it is almost time for your next dose, skip the missed dose and go back to your regular dose. DO NOT take a double dose.

DO NOT keep or use outdated medication. Keep all medication out of the reach of children.

POSSIBLE SIDE EFFECTS:

 Be sure to tell your doctor if the following occur: stomach cramps, loss of appetite, nausea, breast tenderness, swelling of the extremities, abnormal vaginal bleeding, skin rash, chest pain or difficult breathing, severe headache, blurred vision or yellow coloration of the skin or eyes.

PROZAC

THIS MEDICATION IS USED:

To treat depression.

PROPER USE OF THIS MEDICATION:

Take this medicine with a glass of water. If it upsets your stomach you may take it with food.

If you are taking the liquid form, there are special measuring devices available to measure your dose, ask your pharmacist if you want one.

SPECIAL INSTRUCTIONS:

You may experience dizziness, blurred vision or drowsiness from this medicine. If you do, be careful driving or performing hazardous tasks.

Alcoholic beverages can increase the drowsiness.

This medicine may cause lightheadedness. Sit or lie down at the first signs. Avoid sudden changes in posture. Be careful going up and down stairs.

DO NOT take nonprescription cough/cold, hay fever, diet or sleep aid products without asking your doctor or pharmacist.

It may take several weeks before the full effects of this medicine are noticed. DO NOT change the amount of medicine taken nor stop taking it without consulting your doctor.

If you miss a dose of this medicine, take it as soon as possible. But, if it is almost time for your next dose, skip the missed dose and go back to your regular dose. DO NOT take a double dose.

DO NOT keep or use outdated medication. Keep all medication out of the reach of children.

POSSIBLE SIDE EFFECTS:

 Be sure to tell your doctor if the following occur: blurred vision or eye pain, nervousness or confusion, irregular heartbeat or pulse, fainting spells, difficulty getting to sleep or urinating, severe drowsiness, troubled breathing, high fever or hallucinations, excessive sweating or seizures.

PRILOSEC

THIS MEDICATION IS USED:

To treat a number of conditions, including ulcers and other diseases in which the stomach produces too much acid.

PROPER USE OF THIS MEDICATION:

 The best time to take this medicine is before a meal, preferably the morning meal, to reduce the increased stomach acid that occurs after eating.

 This medication should be swallowed whole. DO NOT open, chew or crush the medication.

SPECIAL INSTRUCTIONS:

 Proper control of your condition requires you to take this medicine as instructed at the same time every day, DO NOT skip a dose nor stop taking the medicine without asking your doctor.

You should continue to take this medicine even if you are feeling better to help prevent future stomach pain.

 This medication may be taken with antacids to aid in the relief of pain, unless otherwise instructed by your doctor.

If you miss a dose of this medicine, take it as soon as possible. But, if it is almost time for your next dose, skip the missed dose and go back to your regular dose. DO NOT take a double dose.

DO NOT keep or use outdated medication. Keep all medication out of the reach of children.

POSSIBLE SIDE EFFECTS:

 Be sure to tell your doctor if the following occur: persistent dizziness or headache, skin rash, unusual tiredness or weakness, persistent sore throat or fever, continued abdominal pain or black tarry stools.

BARBITURATE

Amobarbital, Amytal, Butabarbital, Butisol, Mebaral, Nembutal, Pentobarbital, Phenobarbital, Secobarbital, Seconal, Tuinal

THIS MEDICATION IS USED:

For many different medical reasons including to relieve anxiety and tension before surgery, to control some types of seizure disorders or to help you sleep.

PROPER USE OF THIS MEDICATION:

 Take this medicine with a glass of water. If it upsets your stomach you may take it with food.

 If you are taking the liquid form, there are special measuring devices available to measure your dose, ask your pharmacist if you want one.

SPECIAL INSTRUCTIONS:

 You may experience dizziness, blurred vision or drowsiness from this medicine. If you do, be careful driving or performing hazardous tasks.

 Alcoholic beverages can increase the drowsiness.

DO NOT change the amount of medicine taken nor stop taking it without consulting your doctor.

 If you are taking this medication to control seizures, proper control of this condition requires you to take this medicine as instructed at the same time every day, DO NOT skip a dose nor stop taking the medicine without asking your doctor.

If you miss a dose of this medicine, take it as soon as possible. But, if it is almost time for your next dose, skip the missed dose and go back to your regular dose. DO NOT take a double dose.

DO NOT keep or use outdated medication. Keep all medication out of the reach of children.

POSSIBLE SIDE EFFECTS:

Be sure to tell your doctor if the following occur: excessive drowsiness, confusion or depression, difficult breathing, wheezing, unusual heartbeat, excitement, bruising or bleeding, persistent fever or sore throat or yellow coloration of the skin or eyes.

FLUORIDE CONTAINING PRODUCTS

Adiflor, Mulvidren-F, Poly-Vi-Flor, Tri-Vi-Flor, Vi-Daylin/F,
Vitamins (Fluoride Containing)

THIS MEDICATION IS USED:

To reduce the number of cavities in the teeth due to low
fluoride levels in the water supply.

PROPER USE OF THIS MEDICATION:

This medication may be supplied with vitamins or as special dental treatments.

 DO NOT take dairy products or antacids within 1 hour of
this medication.

 If you are taking the chewable tablet form, it should be
chewed well before swallowing. Follow each dose with a
glass of water.

 If you are taking the liquid form, measure the dose using
the measuring device provided with your medication. If
you have any questions about how to measure the dose, ask
your pharmacist.

You may mix this medication with fruit juice or water but
DO NOT mix it with milk.

SPECIAL INSTRUCTIONS:

 It is important that you make regular visits to your dentist
to make sure this medication is working properly.

DO NOT change the amount of medicine taken nor stop
taking it without consulting your doctor.

Always keep this medication in the original plastic container.

If you miss a dose of this medicine, take it as soon as possible. But, if it is almost time for your next dose, skip the
missed dose and go back to your regular dose. DO NOT
take a double dose.

DO NOT keep or use outdated medications. Keep all
medications out of the reach of children.

In case of accidental overdose contact your poison control center immediately.

POSSIBLE SIDE EFFECTS:

 Be sure to tell your doctor if the following occur: black, brown or white spots on your teeth, stiffness, pain and aching of bones, black tarry stools, or severe nausea, vomiting, or diarrhea.

ERYTHROMYCIN/SULFONAMIDE
Erythromycin/Sulfisoxasole, Pediazole

THIS MEDICATION IS USED:

To treat infections.

PROPER USE OF THIS MEDICATION:

 This medication should be taken with a glass of water and it can be taken with or without food.

 This medication should be stored in the refrigerator and used within 14 days. The contents should be shaken well just before measuring the dose. There are special measuring devices available, ask your pharmacist for one.

SPECIAL INSTRUCTIONS:

 The recommended length of treatment is 7-10 days. You should take all the medication unless otherwise instructed by your doctor.

 It is recommended that you drink lots of fluids while you are taking this medication.

 This medicine may make your skin more sensitive to sunlight or sunlamps. Ask your pharmacist about a suitable sunblock product (of at least SPF 15) to minimize problems during exposure.

 If you experience diarrhea while on this medicine, DO NOT take any antidiarrheal medicine without first asking your doctor or pharmacist.

If you miss a dose, take the missed dose as soon as possible. But if it is almost time for your next dose (within 2 hours), DOUBLE that dose. Then go back to your regular dosing schedule.

DO NOT keep or use outdated medication. Keep all medication out of the reach of children.

POSSIBLE SIDE EFFECTS:

 Be sure to tell your doctor if the following occur: skin rash, hives or itching, prolonged nausea, vomiting or diarrhea, sore throat, fever, unusual bleeding or bruising, or yellow coloration of the eyes or skin.

SUPRAX

THIS MEDICATION IS USED:
To treat infections.

PROPER USE OF THIS MEDICATION:

This medicine should be taken with a glass of water and it can be taken with or without food.

If you are taking the liquid form, it may be kept at room temperature. The contents should be shaken well just before measuring the dose. There are special measuring devices available, ask your pharmacist if you want one.

SPECIAL INSTRUCTIONS:

The recommended length of treatment is 7-10 days. You should take all the medication unless otherwise instructed by your doctor.

If you experience diarrhea while taking this medicine, DO NOT take any antidiarrheal medicine without first asking your doctor or pharmacist.

If you miss a dose, take the missed dose as soon as possible. But if it is almost time for your next dose (within 2 hours), space the missed dose and the next dose 10-12 hours apart. Then go back to your regular dosing schedule.

DO NOT keep or use outdated medication. Keep all medication out of the reach of children.

POSSIBLE SIDE EFFECTS:

Be sure to tell your doctor if the following occur: skin rash, hives or itching, shortness of breath or wheezing, swelling of the face, prolonged nausea, vomiting or diarrhea, black tongue, or persistent sore throat or fever.

CORTICOSTEROID (INTRANASAL INHALER)

Beconase Inhaler, Decadron Turbinaire,
Nasacort Inhaler, Vancenase Inhaler

THIS MEDICATION IS USED:

In the nose to relieve or prevent the discomfort of hay fever and other nasal problems.

PROPER USE OF THIS MEDICATION:

Remove the dust cap and shake the canister well before using it.

Gently blow your nose to clear the nostrils just before using this medicine.

 Close one nostril with your finger, tilt head slightly forward and carefully insert the nasal applicator into the open nostril.

Press downward firmly using your middle finger, while using your thumb on the base for support.

Breathe gently inward through the nostril and breathe out through the mouth.

Repeat in other nostril.

Replace the dust cap after use.

SPECIAL INSTRUCTIONS:

 To help prevent contamination from nasal secretions, rinse the applicator in warm water after each use.

 Instructions for each brand of inhaler are similar, but slightly different. Read them carefully and follow the directions. If you have any questions, ask your doctor or pharmacist.

 Proper control of your condition requires you to use this medicine as instructed at the same time every day, DO NOT skip a dose nor stop using the medicine without asking your doctor.

It is important that you continue using this medicine as your doctor has instructed. It may take several days before improvement is noticed.

For the first 2-3 days, if you have excessive nasal congestion, you may use a decongestant nasal spray just prior to using this medication.

If you miss a dose of this medicine, use it as soon as possible. But, if it is almost time for your next dose, skip the missed dose and go back to your regular dose. DO NOT take a double dose.

DO NOT keep or use outdated medicine. Keep this medicine at room temperature, in its original container and out of the reach of children.

POSSIBLE SIDE EFFECTS:

Be sure to tell your doctor if the following occur: continued nasal irritation, excessive sneezing, bloody discharge from the nose, persistent sore throat, swelling of the face, hands or feet, skin rash, difficulty in breathing or muscle cramps or pain.

NITROGLYCERIN OINTMENT

Nitro-Bid Topical, Nitroglycerin Topical, Nitrol Topical, Nitrong Topical, Nitrostat Topical

THIS MEDICATION IS USED:

To prevent angina attacks.

PROPER USE OF THIS MEDICATION:

 This medicine is measured in inches. Apply the prescribed length of ointment to the chest area of the body using the special measuring paper provided by the manufacturer.

DO NOT rub or massage the ointment into the skin; just spread a thin, even layer, covering an area of the same size each time it is applied.

 BEFORE APPLYING a new dose REMOVE any RE-MAINING OINTMENT on the skin from the last dose.

Once the ointment is applied, cover it with a product such as a plastic kitchen wrap and hold in place with adhesive tape. This will enable the ointment to penetrate easier through the skin and also protect your clothing from the ointment.

Change the application site with each administration to avoid skin irritation.

SPECIAL INSTRUCTIONS:

 This medicine may cause lightheadedness. Sit or lie down at the first signs. Avoid sudden changes in posture. Be careful going up and down stairs.

Alcoholic beverages can increase lightheadedness.

 Proper control of your condition requires you to use this medicine as instructed at the same time every day, DO NOT skip a dose nor stop using the medicine without asking your doctor.

If you miss a dose of this medicine, use it as soon as possible. But, if it is almost time for your next dose, skip the

missed dose and go back to your regular dose. DO NOT use a double dose.

DO NOT keep or use outdated medication. Keep all medication out of the reach of children.

POSSIBLE SIDE EFFECTS:

 Be sure to tell your doctor if the following occur: persistent lightheadedness, flushing of the face and neck, headache or a fast pulse.

PEPCID

THIS MEDICATION IS USED:

To treat a number of conditions, including ulcers and other diseases in which the stomach produces too much acid.

PROPER USE OF THIS MEDICATION:

The best time to take this medicine is before meals to reduce the increased stomach acid that occurs after meals. The bedtime dose does not need to be taken with food.

 If you are using antacids, they should be taken 1 hour before or after this medicine.

The liquid form requires the contents to be shaken well just before measuring the dose.

 Discard unused Pepcid liquid after 30 days. There are special measuring devices available, ask your pharmacist if you want one.

SPECIAL INSTRUCTIONS:

 Proper control of your condition requires you to take this medicine as instructed at the same time every day, DO NOT skip a dose nor stop taking the medicine without asking your doctor.

You should continue to take this medicine even if you are feeling better to help prevent future stomach pain.

 You may experience dizziness, blurred vision or drowsiness from this medicine. If you do, be careful driving or performing hazardous tasks.

If you miss a dose of this medicine, take it as soon as possible. But, if it is almost time for your next dose, skip the missed dose and go back to your regular dose. DO NOT take a double dose.

DO NOT keep or use outdated medication. Keep all medication out of the reach of children.

POSSIBLE SIDE EFFECTS:

 Be sure to tell your doctor if the following occur: persistent dizziness or headache, skin rash, confusion or black tarry stools.

CALAN SR - ISOPTIN SR
Verapamil ER

THIS MEDICATION IS USED:

For many conditions, including high blood pressure, angina and irregular heartbeat.

PROPER USE OF THIS MEDICATION:

This medicine should be taken with food.

This is a controlled release form which should be swallowed whole, NOT crushed or chewed.

SPECIAL INSTRUCTIONS:

This medicine may cause lightheadedness. Sit or lie down at the first signs. Avoid sudden changes in posture. Be careful going up and down stairs. Be careful driving or performing hazardous tasks.

The use of alcohol while taking this medicine may increase the chance of dizziness.

Proper control of your condition requires you to take this medicine as instructed at the same time every day, DO NOT skip a dose nor stop taking the medicine without asking your doctor.

Since this medicine does not cure but helps to control your condition, you should continue to take it even if you are feeling well.

DO NOT take nonprescription cough/cold or diet products without asking your doctor or pharmacist.

If you miss a dose of this medicine, take it as soon as possible. But, if it is almost time for your next dose, skip the missed dose and go back to your regular dose. DO NOT take a double dose.

DO NOT keep or use outdated medication. Keep all medication out of the reach of children.

POSSIBLE SIDE EFFECTS:

 Be sure to tell your doctor if the following occur: headache, nausea, swelling of the extremities, unusually slow heartbeat, chest pain, unusual tiredness or difficult breathing.

HISMANAL

THIS MEDICATION IS USED:

To relieve the runny nose, watery eyes and sneezing of colds and hay fever. It also may also be used for allergic reactions.

PROPER USE OF THIS MEDICATION:

 Unless your doctor has told you differently, this medicine should be taken on an empty stomach with a glass of water at least 1 hour before or 2 hours after a meal.

SPECIAL INSTRUCTIONS:

If your mouth becomes dry, you may suck on hard candy, chew gum or use a saliva substitute.

It is important that you take this medicine exactly as your doctor has instructed, DO NOT take more doses than prescribed by your doctor.

 You should NOT take nonprescription cough/cold products without asking your doctor or pharmacist.

You should talk with your doctor before taking the following prescription medications: erythromycin derivatives, ketoconazole (Nizoral), or itraconazole (Sporanox).

 Tell your doctor if you are pregnant, plan to become pregnant or are breastfeeding.

If you miss a dose of this medicine, take it as soon as possible. But, if it is almost time for your next dose, skip the missed dose and go back to your regular dosing schedule. DO NOT take a double dose.

DO NOT keep or use outdated medication. Keep all medication out of the reach of children.

POSSIBLE SIDE EFFECTS:

 Be sure to tell your doctor if the following occur: thickening of the bronchial secretions, headache, dry mouth, blurred vision, drowsiness, increased appetite, nervousness, dizziness, nausea or upset stomach.

ACE INHIBITOR
Accupril, Altace, Lotensin, Prinivil, Vasotec, Zestril

THIS MEDICATION IS USED:

To treat high blood pressure. Some forms are also used to treat congestive heart failure.

PROPER USE OF THIS MEDICATION:

This medicine can be taken with food or on an empty stomach. However, to maintain the proper amount in the body, it is best that each dose either always be taken with food or always be taken on an empty stomach.

SPECIAL INSTRUCTIONS:

This medicine may cause lightheadedness. Sit or lie down at the first signs. Avoid sudden changes in posture. Be careful going up and down stairs. Be careful driving or performing hazardous tasks.

Proper control of your condition requires you to take this medicine as instructed at the same time every day, DO NOT skip a dose nor stop taking the medicine without asking your doctor.

Since this medicine does not cure but helps to control your condition, you should continue to take it even if you are feeling well.

You should not use salt substitutes or take nonprescription cough/cold or diet products without asking your doctor or pharmacist.

If you become pregnant, consult your doctor promptly about switching to a different drug.

If you miss a dose of this medicine, take it as soon as possible. But, if it is almost time for your next dose, skip the missed dose and go back to your regular dose. DO NOT take a double dose.

DO NOT keep or use outdated medicine. Keep this medicine at room temperature, in its original container and out of the reach of children.

POSSIBLE SIDE EFFECTS:

Be sure to tell your doctor if the following occur: persistent sore throat or fever, swelling of the extremities, eyes, lips, face or tongue, difficult breathing, impaired taste, skin rash, nausea or vomiting.

MONOPRIL

THIS MEDICATION IS USED:

 To treat high blood pressure.

PROPER USE OF THIS MEDICATION:

 This medicine can be taken with food or on an empty stomach. However, to maintain the proper amount in the body, it is best that each dose either always be taken with food or always be taken on an empty stomach.

 DO NOT take antacids within 2 hours of taking this medication.

SPECIAL INSTRUCTIONS:

 This medicine may cause lightheadedness. Sit or lie down at the first signs. Avoid sudden changes in posture. Be careful going up and down stairs. Be careful driving or performing hazardous tasks.

 Proper control of your condition requires you to take this medicine as instructed at the same time every day, DO NOT skip a dose nor stop taking the medicine without asking your doctor.

Since this medicine does not cure but helps to control your condition, you should continue to take it even if you are feeling well.

 You should not use salt substitutes or take nonprescription cough/cold or diet products without asking your doctor or pharmacist.

 If you become pregnant, consult your doctor promptly about switching to a different drug.

If you miss a dose of this medicine, take it as soon as possible. But, if it is almost time for your next dose, skip the

missed dose and go back to your regular dose. DO NOT take a double dose.

DO NOT keep or use outdated medicine. Keep this medicine at room temperature, in its original container and out of the reach of children.

POSSIBLE SIDE EFFECTS:

 Be sure to tell your doctor if the following occur: persistent sore throat or fever, swelling of the extremities, eyes, lips, face or tongue, difficult breathing, impaired taste, skin rash, nausea or vomiting.

DIURETIC, POTASSIUM SPARING
Aldactone, Dyrenium, Triamterene

THIS MEDICATION IS USED:

 To help remove excess fluid and salt, decrease swelling and treat high blood pressure.

PROPER USE OF THIS MEDICATION:

You should take this medicine at the same time every day. The best time is before breakfast.

 If stomach upset occurs, you may take this medicine with food unless told otherwise.

SPECIAL INSTRUCTIONS:

 This medicine may cause lightheadedness. Sit or lie down at the first signs. Avoid sudden changes in posture. Be careful going up and down stairs. Be careful driving or performing hazardous tasks.

 Proper control of your condition requires you to take this medicine as instructed at the same time every day, DO NOT skip a dose nor stop taking the medicine without asking your doctor.

Since this medicine does not cure but helps to control your condition, you should continue to take it even if you are feeling well.

 Diet is an important part of managing your blood pressure. You should decrease your sodium intake and not use salt substitutes without asking your doctor or pharmacist.

 DO NOT take nonprescription cough/cold or diet products without asking your doctor or pharmacist.

If you miss a dose of this medicine, take it as soon as possible. But, if it is almost time for your next dose, skip the missed dose and go back to your regular dose. DO NOT take a double dose.

DO NOT keep or use outdated medication. Keep all medication out of the reach of children.

POSSIBLE SIDE EFFECTS:

 Be sure to tell your doctor if the following occur: lightheadedness, nausea or vomiting or muscle weakness or cramps.

AMILORIDE, MIDAMOR

THIS MEDICATION IS USED:

To help remove excess fluid and salt, decrease swelling and treat high blood pressure.

PROPER USE OF THIS MEDICATION:

You should take this medicine at the same time every day. The best time is with breakfast.

SPECIAL INSTRUCTIONS:

This medicine may cause lightheadedness. Sit or lie down at the first signs. Avoid sudden changes in posture. Be careful going up and down stairs. Be careful driving or performing hazardous tasks.

Proper control of your condition requires you to take this medicine as instructed at the same time every day, DO NOT skip a dose nor stop taking the medicine without asking your doctor.

Since this medicine does not cure but helps to control your condition, you should continue to take it even if you are feeling well.

Diet is an important part of managing your blood pressure. You should decrease your sodium intake and not use salt substitutes without asking your doctor or pharmacist.

DO NOT take nonprescription cough/cold or diet products without asking your doctor or pharmacist.

If you miss a dose of this medicine, take it as soon as possible. But, if it is almost time for your next dose, skip the missed dose and go back to your regular dose. DO NOT take a double dose.

DO NOT keep or use outdated medication. Keep all medication out of the reach of children.

POSSIBLE SIDE EFFECTS:

Be sure to tell your doctor if the following occur: light-headedness, nausea or vomiting or muscle weakness or cramps.

POTASSIUM, EFFERVESCENT

K-Lor, K-Lyte, K-Lyte/CL, Kato, Kay Ciel, Klor-Con, Klor-Con/EF, Klorvess Effervescent, Kolyum, Potassium Chloride

THIS MEDICATION IS USED:

As a potassium supplement.

PROPER USE OF THIS MEDICATION:

 Dissolve the tablet or powder in at least a half of glass of water or other fluid. Before drinking the liquid make sure the tablet or powder has completely dissolved then sip the mixture slowly.

 Take this medication with food and a glass of water to help avoid upsetting your stomach.

SPECIAL INSTRUCTIONS:

 You should NOT use salt substitutes without asking your doctor or pharmacist. These products also contain potassium.

 It is recommended that you drink lots of fluids while taking this medication.

It is important that you take this medicine exactly as your doctor has instructed.

If you miss a dose of this medicine, take it as soon as possible. But, if it is almost time for your next dose, skip the missed dose and go back to your regular dose. DO NOT take a double dose.

DO NOT keep or use outdated medication. Keep all medication out of the reach of children.

POSSIBLE SIDE EFFECTS:

 Be sure to tell your doctor if the following occur: irregular heartbeat, unusual tiredness, difficult breathing, mental confusion, numbness or tingling in the extremities, severe vomiting, abdominal pain or black tarry stools.

ANTIHYPERTENSIVE, ALPHA BLOCKER & THIAZIDE
Minizide

THIS MEDICATION IS USED:

To treat high blood pressure.

PROPER USE OF THIS MEDICATION:

This medicine can be taken with or without food.

If stomach upset occurs, you may take this medicine with food.

SPECIAL INSTRUCTIONS:

This medicine may cause you to be drowsy the first few days you take it or when your doctor increases the amount you are taking. If so, be careful driving or performing hazardous tasks.

Alcohol will increase the drowsiness.

This medicine may cause lightheadedness. Sit or lie down at the first signs. Avoid sudden changes in posture. Be careful going up and down stairs.

Proper control of your condition requires you to take this medicine as instructed at the same time every day, DO NOT skip a dose nor stop taking the medicine without asking your doctor.

Since this medicine does not cure but helps to control your condition, you should continue to take it even if you are feeling well.

This medicine may make your skin more sensitive to sunlight or sunlamps. Ask your pharmacist about a suitable sunblock product (of at least SPF 15) to minimize problems during exposure.

DO NOT take nonprescription cough/cold or diet products without asking your doctor or pharmacist

If you miss a dose of this medicine, take it as soon as possible. But, if it is almost time for your next dose, skip the missed dose and go back to your regular dose. DO NOT take a double dose.

DO NOT keep or use outdated medication. Keep all medication out of the reach of children.

POSSIBLE SIDE EFFECTS:

Be sure to tell your doctor if the following occur: skin rash, nausea, chest pain, swelling, dry mouth or yellowing of the skin or eyes.

POTASSIUM, LIQUID

Cena-K, Kaochlor, Kaon, Kaon-CL, Kay Ciel, Klorvess, Kolyum, Potachlor, Potassium Chloride, Potassium Gluconate

THIS MEDICATION IS USED:

As a potassium supplement.

PROPER USE OF THIS MEDICATION:

 Dilute this medicine with at least a half glass of water, fruit juice or other liquid before taking it. This will help reduce the salty taste.

Sip the liquid slowly.

 Take this medication with food and a glass of water to help avoid upsetting your stomach.

There are special measuring devices available to measure your dose, ask your pharmacist if you want one.

SPECIAL INSTRUCTIONS:

 You should NOT use salt substitutes without asking your doctor or pharmacist. These products also contain potassium.

 It is recommended that you drink lots of fluids while taking this medication.

It is important that you take this medicine exactly as your doctor has instructed.

If you miss a dose of this medicine, take it as soon as possible. But, if it is almost time for your next dose, skip the missed dose and go back to your regular dose. DO NOT take a double dose.

DO NOT keep or use outdated medication. Keep all medication out of the reach of children.

POSSIBLE SIDE EFFECTS:

 Be sure to tell your doctor if the following occur: irregular heartbeat, unusual tiredness, difficult breathing, mental confusion, numbness or tingling in the extremities, severe vomiting, abdominal pain or black tarry stools.

AMANTADINE, SYMMETREL

THIS MEDICATION IS USED:

To treat Parkinson's Disease. It is also used to prevent or treat certain flu infections.

PROPER USE OF THIS MEDICATION:

 Take this medicine with a glass of water. If it upsets your stomach you may take it with food.

 If you are taking the liquid form, there are special measuring devices available to measure your dose, ask your pharmacist if you want one.

SPECIAL INSTRUCTIONS:

 You may experience dizziness, blurred vision or drowsiness from this medicine. If you do, be careful driving or performing hazardous tasks.

Alcoholic beverages can increase drowsiness.

 This medicine may cause lightheadedness. Sit or lie down at the first signs. Avoid sudden changes in posture. Be careful going up and down stairs.

 Proper control of your condition requires you to take this medicine as instructed at the same time every day, DO NOT skip a dose nor stop taking the medicine without asking your doctor.

If your mouth becomes dry, you may suck on hard candy, chew gum or use a saliva substitute.

If you miss a dose of this medicine, take it as soon as possible. But, if it is almost time for your next dose, skip the missed dose and go back to your regular dose. DO NOT take a double dose.

DO NOT keep or use outdated medication. Keep all medication out of the reach of children.

POSSIBLE SIDE EFFECTS:

 Be sure to tell your doctor if the following occur: excessive dizziness or lightheadedness, restlessness, irritability, nausea, loss of appetite, nervousness, confusion.

BACLOFEN, LIORESAL

THIS MEDICATION IS USED:

To relieve spasms, cramping and tightness of muscles caused by conditions such as multiple sclerosis or injuries to the spine.

PROPER USE OF THIS MEDICATION:

 Take this medicine with a glass of water. If it upsets your stomach you may take it with food.

SPECIAL INSTRUCTIONS:

 You may experience dizziness, blurred vision or drowsiness from this medicine. If you do, be careful driving or performing hazardous tasks.

Alcoholic beverages can increase the drowsiness.

 This medicine may cause lightheadedness. Sit or lie down at the first signs. Avoid sudden changes in posture. Be careful going up and down stairs.

 Proper control of your condition requires you to take this medicine as instructed at the same time every day, DO NOT skip a dose nor stop taking the medicine without asking your doctor.

If you miss a dose of this medicine, take it as soon as possible. But, if it is almost time for your next dose, skip the missed dose and go back to your regular dose. DO NOT take a double dose.

DO NOT keep or use outdated medication. Keep all medication out of the reach of children.

POSSIBLE SIDE EFFECTS:

 Be sure to tell your doctor if the following occur: nausea or vomiting, difficult breathing, excessive drowsiness, confusion or severe headache.

MUSCLE RELAXANT & ASPIRIN
Norgesic, Norgesic Forte, Robaxisal

THIS MEDICATION IS USED:

To relax muscles and to relieve muscle pain and discomfort.

PROPER USE OF THIS MEDICATION:

Take this medicine with a glass of water. If it upsets your stomach you may take it with food.

SPECIAL INSTRUCTIONS:

 You may experience dizziness, blurred vision or drowsiness from this medicine. Be careful driving or performing hazardous tasks.

Alcoholic beverages can increase the drowsiness.

 This medicine may cause lightheadedness. Sit or lie down at the first signs. Avoid sudden changes in posture. Be careful going up and down stairs.

DO NOT change the amount of medicine taken nor stop taking it without consulting your doctor.

 DO NOT take nonprescription ibuprofen, aspirin or acetaminophen products while taking this drug without checking with your doctor or pharmacist.

 If taken for a few days, you may experience some constipation. You should increase the amount of bulk in your diet (bran, psyllium, and fresh fruits) and drink lots of fluids.

 Discard doses that have a strong vinegar odor. The aspirin has decomposed.

If you miss a dose of this medicine, take it as soon as possible. But, if it is almost time for your next dose, skip the missed dose and go back to your regular dose. DO NOT take a double dose.

DO NOT keep or use outdated medication. Keep all medication out of the reach of children.

POSSIBLE SIDE EFFECTS:

 Be sure to tell your doctor if the following occur: nausea, troubled breathing, skin rash, blurred vision, severe headache, persistent sore throat or fever, irregular heartbeat, yellow coloration of the skin or eyes, ringing or buzzing in the ears or black, tarry stools.

ANTIHYPERTENSIVE, ALPHA STIMULANT & THIAZIDE

Aldoril, Aldoril-D, Clonidine/Chlorthalidone, Combipres

THIS MEDICATION IS USED:

To treat high blood pressure.

PROPER USE OF THIS MEDICATION:

This medication should be taken with a glass of water and it can be taken with or without food.

If it upsets your stomach, take it with food.

SPECIAL INSTRUCTIONS:

This medicine may cause you to be drowsy the first few days you take it or when your doctor increases the amount you are taking. If it does, be careful driving or performing hazardous tasks. Alcoholic beverages will increase the drowsiness.

This medicine may cause lightheadedness. Sit or lie down at the first signs. Avoid sudden changes in posture. Be careful going up and down stairs.

Proper control of your condition requires you to take this medicine as instructed at the same time every day, DO NOT skip a dose nor stop taking the medicine without asking your doctor.

Since this medicine does not cure but helps to control your condition, you should continue to take it even if you are feeling well.

DO NOT take nonprescription cough/cold or diet products without asking your doctor or pharmacist.

This medicine may make your skin more sensitive to sunlight or sunlamps. Ask your pharmacist about a suitable sunblock product (of at least SPF 15) to minimize problems during exposure.

If you miss a dose of this medicine, take it as soon as possible. But, if it is almost time for your next dose, skip the missed dose and go back to your regular dose. DO NOT take a double dose.

DO NOT keep or use outdated medication. Keep all medication out of the reach of children.

POSSIBLE SIDE EFFECTS:

 Be sure to tell your doctor if the following occur: changes in moods, nausea, chest pain, unusual swelling or yellow coloration of the skin.

PHENOTHIAZINE, ANTIEMETIC
Compazine, Compazine Spansule, Phenergan, Prochlorperazine, Promethazine, Tigan, Trimethobenzamide

THIS MEDICATION IS USED:

To relieve or prevent motion sickness, nausea, vomiting and dizziness. It is also used to help some people sleep.

PROPER USE OF THIS MEDICATION:

 Take this medicine with a glass of water. If it upsets your stomach you may take it with food.

 If you are taking the liquid form, there are special measuring devices available to measure your dose, ask your pharmacist if you want one.

SPECIAL INSTRUCTIONS:

 You may experience dizziness, blurred vision or drowsiness from this medicine. Be careful driving or performing hazardous tasks.

Alcoholic beverages can increase the drowsiness.

 This medicine may cause lightheadedness. Sit or lie down at the first signs. Avoid sudden changes in posture. Be careful going up and down stairs.

DO NOT change the amount of medicine taken nor stop taking it without consulting your doctor.

 This medicine may make your skin more sensitive to sunlight or sunlamps. Ask your pharmacist about a suitable sunblock product (of at least SPF 15) to minimize problems during exposure.

If you miss a dose of this medicine, take it as soon as possible. But, if it is almost time for your next dose, skip the missed dose and go back to your regular dose. DO NOT take a double dose.

DO NOT keep or use outdated medication. Keep all medication out of the reach of children.

POSSIBLE SIDE EFFECTS:

 Be sure to tell your doctor if the following occur: skin rash, persistent sore throat or fever, blurred vision, yellow coloration of the skin or eyes, uncontrollable trembling of the extremities or muscle spasms of the neck or back.

ANTIEMETIC, SUPPOSITORY
Compazine, Phenergan, Prochlorperazine, Promethazine, Thorazine, Tigan, Trimethobenzamide

THIS MEDICATION IS USED:

To relieve or prevent motion sickness, nausea, vomiting and dizziness.

PROPER USE OF THIS MEDICATION:

Remove the wrapper. Holding the blunt end, moisten the suppository with lukewarm water.

If the suppository is too soft to insert run cold water over it before removing the wrapper.

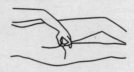

Lie down on your side and push the pointed end first, just inside the rectum.

SPECIAL INSTRUCTIONS:

You may experience dizziness, blurred vision or drowsiness from this medicine. Be careful driving or performing hazardous tasks.

Alcoholic beverages can increase the drowsiness.

This medicine may cause lightheadedness. Sit or lie down at the first signs. Avoid sudden changes in posture. Be careful going up and down stairs.

DO NOT change the amount of medicine used nor stop using it without consulting your doctor.

This medicine may make your skin more sensitive to sunlight or sunlamps. Ask your pharmacist about a suitable sunblock product (of at least SPF 15) to minimize problems during exposure.

DO NOT keep or use outdated medication. Keep all medication out of the reach of children.

POSSIBLE SIDE EFFECTS:

 Be sure to tell your doctor if the following occur: skin rash, persistent sore throat or fever, blurred vision, yellow coloration of the skin or eyes, uncontrollable trembling of the extremities or muscle spasms of the neck or back.

PHENAZOPYRIDINE

Geridium, Phenazodine, Phenazopyridine, Pyridiate, Pyridium, Urodine, Urogesic

THIS MEDICATION IS USED:

To relieve the pain, burning and discomfort caused by infection or irritation of the urinary tract.

PROPER USE OF THIS MEDICATION:

Take this medication with food and a glass of water to avoid upsetting your stomach.

SPECIAL INSTRUCTIONS:

Length of treatment should not exceed 2 days unless otherwise instructed by your doctor.

If you are a diabetic, this medicine may interfere with urine test for sugar or ketones. Report any abnormal results to your doctor before changing the dose of insulin or oral antidiabetic drugs.

This medicine will cause the urine to change color to a reddish orange. DO NOT be alarmed, because this is normal.

If you miss a dose of this medicine, take it as soon as possible. But, if it is almost time for your next dose, skip the missed dose and go back to your regular dosing schedule. DO NOT take a double dose.

DO NOT keep or use outdated medication. Keep all medication out of the reach of children.

POSSIBLE SIDE EFFECTS:

Be sure to tell your doctor if the following occur: skin rash, unusual tiredness or weakness, headache, indigestion, stomach pain or cramps, or yellow coloration of the eyes or skin.

GRISEOFULVIN
Fulvicin P/G, Fulvicin U/F, Grifulvin V, Gris-Peg, Grisactin, Grisactin Ultra

THIS MEDICATION IS USED:

To treat fungus infections of the skin, hair, fingernails and toenails.

PROPER USE OF THIS MEDICATION:

 To maximize absorption and to reduce the chance of stomach upset, this medicine SHOULD be taken with food.

 If you are taking the liquid form the contents should be shaken well just before measuring the dose. There are special measuring devices available, ask your pharmacist if you want one.

SPECIAL INSTRUCTIONS:

 Long term therapy is needed (possibly 6 months or longer). It is important to take the full length of treatment unless otherwise instructed by your doctor.

 This medicine may make your skin more sensitive to sunlight or sunlamps. Ask your pharmacist about a suitable sunblock product (of at least SPF 15) to minimize problems during exposure.

If you miss a dose of this medicine, take it as soon as possible. But, if it is almost time for your next dose, skip the missed dose and go back to your regular dosing schedule. DO NOT take a double dose.

DO NOT keep or use outdated medication. Keep all medication out of the reach of children.

POSSIBLE SIDE EFFECTS:

 Be sure to tell your doctor if the following occur: recurrent sore throat or fever, dizziness, drowsiness or confusion, tingling or pain in the extremities, irritation to the mouth and stomach pain.

CARBONIC ANHYDRASE INHIBITOR
Acetazolamide, Diamox, Diamox Sequels

THIS MEDICATION IS USED:

To treat glaucoma. This medicine is also used to help control certain seizures and treat edema.

PROPER USE OF THIS MEDICATION:

 Take this medicine with a glass of water. If it upsets your stomach you may take it with food.

 The controlled release forms should be swallowed whole, NOT crushed, chewed, or broken.

SPECIAL INSTRUCTIONS:

 A few people may experience dizziness, blurred vision or drowsiness from this medicine. If any of these happen to you, be careful driving or performing hazardous tasks.

 This medicine may cause lightheadedness. Sit or lie down at the first signs. Avoid sudden changes in posture. Be careful going up and down stairs.

 Proper control of your condition requires you to take this medicine as instructed at the same time every day, DO NOT skip a dose nor stop taking the medicine without asking your doctor.

 DO NOT take nonprescription cough/cold, hay fever or sleep aid products without asking your doctor or pharmacist.

If you miss a dose of this medicine, take it as soon as possible. But, if it is almost time for your next dose, skip the missed dose and go back to your regular dose. DO NOT take a double dose.

DO NOT keep or use outdated medication. Keep all medication out of the reach of children.

POSSIBLE SIDE EFFECTS:

Be sure to tell your doctor if the following occur: loss of appetite, persistent gastric pain, flu-like symptoms or tingling, pain or tremors of the extremities.

NOROXIN

THIS MEDICATION IS USED:

To treat infections.

PROPER USE OF THIS MEDICATION:

 This medication should be taken on an empty stomach, either one hour before or two hours after a meal.

 DO NOT take antacids or iron supplements within 2 hours of taking this medication.

SPECIAL INSTRUCTIONS:

 The recommended length of treatment is 7-10 days. You should take all the medication unless otherwise instructed by your doctor.

 It is recommended that you drink lots of fluids while you are taking this medication.

 You may experience dizziness, blurred vision or drowsiness from this medicine. If you do, be careful driving or performing hazardous tasks.

 This medicine may make your skin more sensitive to sunlight or sunlamps. Ask your pharmacist about a suitable sunblock product (of at least SPF 15) to minimize problems during exposure.

Stop this medicine at the first sign of a skin rash or other allergic reaction and tell your doctor.

Be careful taking products containing caffeine while on this medicine, as there may be increased caffeine-related stimulation.

If you miss a dose of this medicine, take it as soon as possible. But, if it is almost time for your next dose, skip the missed dose and go back to your regular dosing schedule.

DO NOT take a double dose.

DO NOT keep or use outdated medication. Keep all medication out of the reach of children.

POSSIBLE SIDE EFFECTS:

 Be sure to tell your doctor if the following occur: skin rash, nausea or vomiting, headache, diarrhea, blurred vision, dizziness or drowsiness, stomach pain or dry mouth.

VALPROIC ACID
Depakene, Depakote

THIS MEDICATION IS USED:

To control convulsions and seizures.

PROPER USE OF THIS MEDICATION:

Take this medicine with a glass of water. If it upsets your stomach you may take it with food.

The controlled release forms should be swallowed whole, NOT crushed or chewed.

If you are taking the liquid form, there are special measuring devices available to measure your dose, ask your pharmacist if you want one.

Some capsule forms of this medication can be swallowed whole or opened up and the contents mixed with food.

SPECIAL INSTRUCTIONS:

You may experience dizziness, blurred vision or drowsiness from this medicine. If you do, be careful driving or performing hazardous tasks.

Alcoholic beverages can increase the drowsiness.

Proper control of your condition requires you to take this medicine as instructed at the same time every day, DO NOT skip a dose nor stop taking the medicine without asking your doctor.

If you miss a dose of this medicine, take it as soon as possible. But, if it is almost time for your next dose, skip the missed dose and go back to your regular dose. DO NOT take a double dose.

DO NOT keep or use outdated medication. Keep all medication out of the reach of children.

POSSIBLE SIDE EFFECTS:

 Be sure to tell your doctor if the following occur: nausea or vomiting, diarrhea, indigestion, blurred vision or unusual bleeding or bruising.

ACE INHIBITOR & THIAZIDE

Prinzide, Vaseretic, Zestoretic

THIS MEDICATION IS USED:

 To treat high blood pressure.

PROPER USE OF THIS MEDICATION:

 This medicine can be taken with food or on an empty stomach. However, to maintain the proper amount in the body, it is best that each dose either always be taken with food or always be taken on an empty stomach.

SPECIAL INSTRUCTIONS:

 This medicine may cause lightheadedness. Sit or lie down at the first signs. Avoid sudden changes in posture. Be careful going up and down stairs.

 Proper control of your condition requires you to take this medicine as instructed at the same time every day, DO NOT skip a dose nor stop taking the medicine without asking your doctor.

Since this medicine does not cure but helps to control your condition, you should continue to take it even if you are feeling well.

 This medicine may make your skin more sensitive to sunlight or sunlamps. Ask your pharmacist about a suitable sunblock product (of at least SPF 15) to minimize problems during exposure.

 You should NOT use salt substitutes or take nonprescription cough/cold or diet products without asking your doctor or pharmacist.

 If you become pregnant, consult your doctor promptly about switching to a different drug.

If you miss a dose of this medicine, take it as soon as possible. But, if it is almost time for your next dose, skip the missed dose and go back to your regular dose. DO NOT take a double dose.

DO NOT keep or use outdated medicine. Keep this medicine at room temperature, in its original container and out of the reach of children.

POSSIBLE SIDE EFFECTS:

 Be sure to tell your doctor if the following occur: persistent sore throat, swelling of the extremities, eyes, lips, face or tongue, difficult breathing, nausea or vomiting, skin rash or yellow coloration of skin.

CAPOZIDE

THIS MEDICATION IS USED:

 To treat high blood pressure.

PROPER USE OF THIS MEDICATION:

 This medication should be taken one hour before meals.

SPECIAL INSTRUCTIONS:

 This medicine may cause lightheadedness. Sit or lie down at the first signs. Avoid sudden changes in posture. Be careful going up and down stairs.

 Proper control of your condition requires you to take this medicine as instructed at the same time every day, DO NOT skip a dose nor stop taking the medicine without asking your doctor.

Since this medicine does not cure but helps to control your condition, you should continue to take it even if you are feeling well.

 This medicine may make your skin more sensitive to sunlight or sunlamps. Ask your pharmacist about a suitable sunblock product (of at least SPF 15) to minimize problems during exposure.

 You should NOT use salt substitutes or take nonprescription cough/cold or diet products without asking your doctor or pharmacist.

 If you become pregnant, consult your doctor promptly about switching to a different drug.

If you miss a dose of this medicine, take it as soon as possible. But, if it is almost time for your next dose, skip the missed dose and go back to your regular dose. DO NOT take a double dose.

DO NOT keep or use outdated medicine. Keep this medicine at room temperature, in its original container and out of the reach of children.

POSSIBLE SIDE EFFECTS:

 Be sure to tell your doctor if the following occur: persistent sore throat, swelling of the extremities, eyes, lips, face or tongue, difficult breathing, nausea or vomiting, skin rash or yellow coloration of skin.

BETA BLOCKER & THIAZIDE

Atenolol w/Chlorthalidone, Corzide, Inderide, Inderide LA,
Lopressor HCT, Normozide, Tenoretic, Timolide

THIS MEDICATION IS USED:

 To treat high blood pressure.

PROPER USE OF THIS MEDICATION:

 This medicine can be taken with food or on an empty stomach. However, to maintain the proper amount in the body, it is best that each dose either always be taken with food or always be taken on an empty stomach.

 The controlled release forms should be swallowed whole, NOT crushed or chewed.

SPECIAL INSTRUCTIONS:

 This medicine may cause lightheadedness. Sit or lie down at the first signs. Avoid sudden changes in posture. Be careful going up and down stairs. Be careful driving or performing hazardous tasks.

 Proper control of your condition requires you to take this medicine as instructed at the same time every day, DO NOT skip a dose nor stop taking the medicine without asking your doctor.

Since this medicine does not cure but helps to control your condition, you should continue to take it even if you are feeling well.

 This medicine may make your skin more sensitive to sunlight or sunlamps. Ask your pharmacist about a suitable sunblock product (of at least SPF 15) to minimize problems during exposure.

 DO NOT take nonprescription cough/cold or diet products without asking your doctor or pharmacist.

If you miss a dose of this medicine, take it as soon as possible. But, if it is almost time for your next dose, skip the missed dose and go back to your regular dose. DO NOT take a double dose.

DO NOT keep or use outdated medication. Keep all medication out of the reach of children.

POSSIBLE SIDE EFFECTS:

Be sure to tell your doctor if the following occur: unusually slow pulse or slow irregular heartbeat, difficult breathing, weakness, muscle cramps or yellow coloration of the eyes or skin.

BUSPAR

THIS MEDICATION IS USED:

To relieve anxiety.

PROPER USE OF THIS MEDICATION:

 Take this medicine with a glass of water. If it upsets your stomach you may take it with food.

SPECIAL INSTRUCTIONS:

 You may experience dizziness, blurred vision or drowsiness from this medicine. If you do, be careful driving or performing hazardous tasks.

Alcoholic beverages can increase the drowsiness.

 This medicine may cause lightheadedness. Sit or lie down at the first signs. Avoid sudden changes in posture. Be careful going up and down stairs.

 Proper control of your condition requires you to take this medicine as instructed at the same time every day, DO NOT skip a dose nor stop taking the medicine without asking your doctor.

It is important that you continue taking this medicine as your doctor has instructed. It may take several days before improvement is noticed.

If you miss a dose of this medicine, take it as soon as possible. But, if it is almost time for your next dose, skip the missed dose and go back to your regular dose. DO NOT take a double dose.

DO NOT keep or use outdated medication. Keep all medication out of the reach of children.

POSSIBLE SIDE EFFECTS:

 Be sure to tell your doctor if the following occur: persistent fever or sore throat, mouth sores, difficult breathing, irregular heartbeat or yellow coloration of the skin or eyes.

ACCUTANE

THIS MEDICATION IS USED:

To treat severe acne.

PROPER USE OF THIS MEDICATION:

 To maximize absorption and reduce the chance of stomach upset, take this medicine with food.

 Swallow this medication WHOLE. DO NOT crush, chew, grind, or break the capsule.

SPECIAL INSTRUCTIONS:

 A detailed leaflet is available with your prescription. Read it and follow its instructions. If you have any questions or need help understanding it, ask your doctor or pharmacist.

DO NOT take vitamin A supplements without contacting your doctor.

 This drug causes severe birth defects. Sexually active women of childbearing age MUST discuss the use of some method of birth control while taking it. Talk to your doctor about this before beginning therapy.

If there is a chance that pregnancy has occurred stop taking this medication and call your doctor right away.

Worsening of your condition may occur during the beginning of therapy. This does not mean that the medicine is not working. DO NOT change the amount of medicine taken nor stop taking it without consulting your doctor.

You may experience decreased night vision while taking this medication. Be careful driving or performing hazardous tasks at night.

 This medicine makes your skin more sensitive to sunlight or sunlamps. Ask your pharmacist about a suitable sunblock product (of at least SPF 15) to minimize problems during exposure.

This drug usually causes dry skin. Ask your pharmacist for a suitable moisturizer.

DO NOT donate blood for transfusion for at least 30 days after stopping this medicine.

DO NOT keep or use outdated medication. Keep all medication out of the reach of children.

POSSIBLE SIDE EFFECTS:

 Be sure to tell your doctor if the following occur: visual disturbances, severe stomach pain or diarrhea, rectal bleeding or severe headache.

BUTALBITAL & ACETAMINOPHEN
Esgic, Fioricet

THIS MEDICATION IS USED:

To treat tension headaches.

PROPER USE OF THIS MEDICATION:

 Take this medication with food and a glass of water to avoid upsetting your stomach.

SPECIAL INSTRUCTIONS:

 You may experience dizziness, blurred vision or drowsiness from this medicine. Be careful driving or performing hazardous tasks.

 Alcoholic beverages can increase the drowsiness.

DO NOT change the amount of medicine taken nor stop taking it without consulting your doctor.

 DO NOT take nonprescription ibuprofen, aspirin or acetaminophen products while taking this drug without checking with your doctor or pharmacist.

If you miss a dose of this medicine, take it as soon as possible. But, if it is almost time for your next dose, skip the missed dose and go back to your regular dose. DO NOT take a double dose.

DO NOT keep or use outdated medication. Keep all medication out of the reach of children.

POSSIBLE SIDE EFFECTS:

 Be sure to tell your doctor if the following occur: difficulty in breathing, severe headache or stomach cramps, persistent sore throat or fever or yellow coloration of the skin or eyes.

ANTIHISTAMINE & DECONGESTANT & NARCOTIC

Actifed w/Codeine, Codimal DH, Codimal PH, Dihistine DH, Dimetane-DC, Endal HD, Myphetane DC, Novahistine DH, Phenergan VC w/Codeine, Phenhist DH, Polyhistine CS, Promethazine VC w/Codeine, Rutuss w/Hydrocodone, Tussar SF, Tussar-2, Vanex HD

THIS MEDICATION IS USED:

To relieve coughing, runny nose, watery eyes, sneezing and stuffiness of colds or hay fever.

PROPER USE OF THIS MEDICATION:

 Take this medicine with a glass of water. If it upsets your stomach you may take it with food.

 If you are taking the liquid form, there are special measuring devices available to measure your dose, ask your pharmacist if you want one.

SPECIAL INSTRUCTIONS:

 You may experience dizziness, blurred vision or drowsiness from this medicine. If you do, be careful driving or performing hazardous tasks.

Alcoholic beverages can increase the drowsiness.

 DO NOT take nonprescription cough/cold, hay fever or sleep aid products without asking your doctor or pharmacist.

If your mouth becomes dry, you may suck on hard candy, chew gum, use a saliva substitute.

 This medicine may make your skin more sensitive to sunlight or sunlamps. Ask your pharmacist about a suitable sunblock product (of at least SPF 15) to minimize problems during exposure.

 If taken for a few days, you may experience some constipation. You should increase the amount of bulk in your diet (bran, psyllium, and fresh fruits) and drink lots of fluids.

If you miss a dose of this medicine, take it as soon as possible. But, if it is almost time for your next dose, skip the missed dose and go back to your regular dose. DO NOT take a double dose.

DO NOT keep or use outdated medicine. Keep this medicine at room temperature, in its original container and out of the reach of children.

POSSIBLE SIDE EFFECTS:

Be sure to tell your doctor if the following occur: drowsiness, blurred vision, dry mouth, headache, mental confusion, loss of appetite, nervousness, chest pain or irregular heartbeat.

ANTIHISTAMINE & DECONGESTANT & NON-NARCOTIC

Carbodec DM, Cardec DM, Dimetane-DX, Myphetane DX, Polyhistine DM, Rondec-DM, Rynatuss, Tussafed

THIS MEDICATION IS USED:

To relieve coughing, runny nose, watery eyes, sneezing and stuffiness of colds or hay fever.

PROPER USE OF THIS MEDICATION:

 Take this medicine with a glass of water. If it upsets your stomach you may take it with food.

Some of the liquid forms require the contents to be shaken well just before measuring the dose.

 There are special measuring devices available, ask your pharmacist if you want one.

SPECIAL INSTRUCTIONS:

 You may experience dizziness, blurred vision or drowsiness from this medicine. If you do, be careful driving or performing hazardous tasks.

Alcoholic beverages can increase drowsiness.

 It is recommended that you drink lots of fluids while you are taking this medication.

 DO NOT take nonprescription cough/cold, hay fever or sleep aid products without asking your doctor or pharmacist.

If your mouth becomes dry, you may suck on hard candy, chew gum or use a saliva substitute.

 This medicine may make your skin more sensitive to sunlight or sunlamps. Ask your pharmacist about a suitable sunblock product (of at least SPF 15) to minimize problems during exposure.

If you miss a dose of this medicine, take it as soon as possible. But, if it is almost time for your next dose, skip the missed dose and go back to your regular dose. DO NOT take a double dose.

DO NOT keep or use outdated medicine. Keep this medicine at room temperature, in its original container and out of the reach of children.

POSSIBLE SIDE EFFECTS:

 Be sure to tell your doctor if the following occur: drowsiness, blurred vision, dry mouth, headache, mental confusion, loss of appetite, nervousness, chest pain or irregular heartbeat.

CHOLYBAR

THIS MEDICATION IS USED:

For a number of conditions including lowering high cholesterol levels in the blood and removing high levels of bile acids due to liver problems.

PROPER USE OF THIS MEDICATION:

Chew each bite of the bar well before swallowing.

Follow each bar (dose) with a glass of water.

SPECIAL INSTRUCTIONS:

You should follow a standard cholesterol lowering diet while taking this medicine. Your diet is the MOST important part of controlling your condition and is necessary if the medicine is to work properly.

Proper control of your condition requires you to take this medicine as instructed at the same time every day, DO NOT skip a dose nor stop taking the medicine without asking your doctor.

This medicine may change the effect of other medicines you are taking. It should be taken 1 hour after or 4 hours before other medications.

It is recommended that you drink lots of fluids while you are taking this medication.

If you miss a dose of this medicine, take it as soon as possible. But, if it is almost time for your next dose, skip the missed dose and go back to your regular dose. DO NOT take a double dose.

DO NOT keep or use outdated medication. Keep all medication out of the reach of children.

POSSIBLE SIDE EFFECTS:

Be sure to tell your doctor if the following occur: constipation, nausea or stomach discomfort.

PRAVACHOL, ZOCOR

THIS MEDICATION IS USED:

To lower levels of cholesterol in the blood.

PROPER USE OF THIS MEDICATION:

This medication may be taken without regards to meals. It should be taken at bedtime.

If it upsets your stomach, take it with food.

SPECIAL INSTRUCTIONS:

You should follow a standard cholesterol lowering diet while taking this medicine. Your diet is the MOST important part of controlling your condition and is necessary if the medicine is to work properly.

DO NOT stop or change the amount of medicine taken without first consulting your doctor.

If you miss a dose of this medicine, take it as soon as possible. But, if it is almost time for your next dose, skip the missed dose and go back to your regular dosing schedule. DO NOT take a double dose.

DO NOT keep or use outdated medication. Keep all medication out of the reach of children.

POSSIBLE SIDE EFFECTS:

Be sure to tell your doctor if the following occur: blurred vision, muscle pain, tenderness or weakness, tiredness, fever, stomach pain, headache, nausea or skin rash.

MINOCYCLINE, MINOCIN

THIS MEDICATION IS USED:

To treat infections.

PROPER USE OF THIS MEDICATION:

 Unless your doctor has told you differently, this medicine should be taken on an empty stomach with a glass of water. You may take it with food if it upsets your stomach.

If you are taking the liquid form, it should be stored at room temperature. The contents should be shaken well just before measuring the dose. There are special measuring devices available, ask your pharmacist if you want one.

The contents of the pellet form should NOT be crushed or chewed.

 DO NOT take antacids or iron supplements within 2 hours of taking this medication.

SPECIAL INSTRUCTIONS:

 The recommended length of treatment is 7-10 days. You should take all the medication unless otherwise instructed by your doctor.

 This medication may make your skin more sensitive to sunlight or sunlamps. Ask your pharmacist about a suitable sunblock product (of at least SPF 15) to reduce exposure problems.

If you miss a dose, take the missed dose as soon as possible. But if it is almost time for your next dose (within 2 hours), DOUBLE that dose. Then go back to your regular dosing schedule.

 This medication may cause dizziness or lightheadedness. If it does, be careful driving or performing hazardous tasks.

DO NOT keep or use outdated medication. Keep all medication out of the reach of children.

POSSIBLE SIDE EFFECTS:

 Be sure to tell your doctor if the following occur: cramps, nausea or vomiting, rectal itch or sores on the tongue or mouth.

BRONCHODILATOR, INHALER
Alupent, Brethaire, Maxair, Metaprel,
Proventil, Tornalate, Ventolin

THIS MEDICATION IS USED:

To treat the symptoms of bronchial asthma, chronic bronchitis and emphysema.

PROPER USE OF THIS MEDICATION:

 If you have any questions concerning how to use your medicine be sure to ask your doctor or pharmacist.

HOW TO USE ORAL INHALERS:

BE SURE the canister is properly inserted into the inhaler unit.

 REMOVE dust cap and SHAKE the can WELL.

Unless your doctor has told you otherwise, exhale fully and place mouthpiece into your mouth with your lips closed around it and your tongue flat.

As you take a deep breath, squeeze the can and mouthpiece together at exactly the same time.

Continue taking a deep breath and hold it for as long as comfortable.

Exhale slowly keeping your lips nearly closed.

 Be sure to wait the prescribed amount of time before inhaling a second dose.

 Notify your doctor if shortness of breath persists after the dose, or, if the dose fails to provide the usual relief.

The dry mouth, which occurs in some patients, can be cared for by rinsing your mouth with water or a mouthwash after the dose.

KEEP THE MOUTHPIECE CLEAN. After each use separate the mouthpiece from the medication canister and rinse the mouthpiece with warm water. DO NOT WIPE.

When not using the inhaler, store it with the dust cap on the mouthpiece. This will prevent dirt and dust from getting into the mouthpiece.

SPECIAL INSTRUCTIONS:

Proper control of your condition requires you to take this medicine as instructed at the same time every day, DO NOT skip a dose nor stop taking the medicine without asking your doctor.

DO NOT take nonprescription cough/cold, hay fever or sleep aid products without asking your doctor or pharmacist.

Instructions for each brand of inhaler are similar, but slightly different. Read them carefully and follow the directions. If you have any questions, ask your doctor or pharmacist.

Cigarette smoking will affect your condition. DO NOT increase the amount of cigarettes you smoke. Instead, try to quit smoking, your doctor or pharmacist can explain various methods.

If you miss a dose of this medicine, take it as soon as possible. But, if it is almost time for your next dose, skip the missed dose and go back to your regular dose. DO NOT take a double dose.

DO NOT keep or use outdated medicine. Keep this medicine at room temperature, in its original container and out of the reach of children.

POSSIBLE SIDE EFFECTS:

Be sure to tell your doctor if the following occur: chest pain, severe dizziness or headache, irregular or pounding heartbeat.

ESTRADERM

THIS MEDICATION IS USED:

For several different medical reasons, including alleviating the symptoms of menopause.

PROPER USE OF THIS MEDICATION:

Wash and dry hands before starting and after applying a patch.

Apply a new patch twice weekly to a clean, dry area of the skin on the trunk of your body, preferably the abdomen.

PLEASE NOTE

The patch SHOULD NOT be applied to the chest or breasts. The waistline is NOT considered a good site of application since tight fitting clothes may rub the patch off.

Apply each new patch to a different skin area.

Apply the patch firmly and hold in place with the palm of your hand for about 10 seconds. Make sure the edges of the patch are in contact with the skin. REMOVE OLD PATCH.

The patch can be worn while you bathe or shower.

If the patch falls off, you may reapply it to the same place. The patch can be held on with adhesive tape.

If a new patch must be used, you should remain on your normal twice weekly schedule.

SPECIAL INSTRUCTIONS:

A detailed leaflet is available with your prescription. Read it and follow its instructions. If you have any questions or need help understanding it, ask your doctor or pharmacist.

If there is a chance that pregnancy has occurred stop using this medication and call your doctor right away.

If you miss a dose of this medication, use it as soon as possible. But, if it is almost time for your next dose, skip the

missed dose and go back to your regular dosing schedule.
DO NOT use a double dose.

DO NOT keep or use outdated medication. Keep all medication out of the reach of children.

POSSIBLE SIDE EFFECTS:

Be sure to tell your doctor if the following occur: any irregular bleeding, breast tenderness, enlargement or lumps, pain or heaviness in the legs or chest, severe headache, dizziness or changes in vision or skin redness or rash.

CYTOTEC

THIS MEDICATION IS USED:

To prevent gastric ulcers in patients on aspirin or nonsteroidal anti-inflammatory drug therapy.

PROPER USE OF THIS MEDICATION:

Take this medication with food and a glass of water to help avoid upset stomach and diarrhea.

SPECIAL INSTRUCTIONS:

A detailed leaflet from the manufacturer is available for your prescription. Read it and follow its instructions. If you have any questions or need help understanding it, ask your doctor or pharmacist.

DO NOT take this medication if you are pregnant and DO NOT become pregnant while taking it.

Sexually active women of childbearing age MUST discuss the use of some method of birth control while taking this medication. Talk to your doctor about this before beginning therapy.

If there is a chance that pregnancy has occurred stop taking this medication and call your doctor right away.

It is important that you take this medicine exactly as your doctor has instructed. DO NOT change the amount of medicine to be taken without first consulting your doctor.

If you experience diarrhea, DO NOT take any antidiarrheal medicine while taking this medicine without first asking your doctor or pharmacist. The diarrhea should stop in a few days. If it does not, contact your doctor.

If you miss a dose of this medicine, take it as soon as possible. But, if it is almost time for your next dose, skip the missed dose and go back to your regular dose. DO NOT take a double dose.

DO NOT keep or use outdated medicine. Keep this medicine at room temperature, in its original container and out of the reach of children.

POSSIBLE SIDE EFFECTS:

 Be sure to tell your doctor if the following occur: prolonged or severe diarrhea, stomach cramps, or nausea or vomiting.

BIAXIN

THIS MEDICATION IS USED:

To treat infections.

PROPER USE OF THIS MEDICATION:

 This medication should be taken with a glass of water and it can be taken with or without food.

SPECIAL INSTRUCTIONS:

 The recommended length of treatment is 7-14 days. You should take all the medication unless otherwise instructed by your doctor.

 If you experience diarrhea while taking this medicine, DO NOT take any antidiarrheal medicine without first asking your doctor or pharmacist.

If you miss a dose, take the missed dose as soon as possible. But if it is almost time for your next dose, space the missed dose and the next dose 5-6 hours apart. Then go back to your regular dosing schedule.

DO NOT keep or use outdated medication. Keep all medication out of the reach of children.

POSSIBLE SIDE EFFECTS:

 Be sure to tell your doctor if the following occur: prolonged or severe nausea, vomiting or diarrhea.

ZOLOFT

THIS MEDICATION IS USED:

To treat depression.

PROPER USE OF THIS MEDICATION:

 Take this medicine with a glass of water. If it upsets your stomach you may take it with food.

SPECIAL INSTRUCTIONS:

 It is possible you may experience dizziness, blurred vision or drowsiness from this medicine. Be careful driving or performing hazardous tasks.

Alcoholic beverages may increase the drowsiness.

 This medicine may cause lightheadedness. Sit or lie down at the first signs. Avoid sudden changes in posture. Be careful going up and down stairs.

 DO NOT take nonprescription cough/cold, hay fever, diet or sleep aid products without asking your doctor or pharmacist.

 It may take several weeks before the full effects of this medicine are noticed. DO NOT change the amount of medicine taken nor stop taking it without consulting your doctor.

If your mouth becomes dry, you may suck on hard candy, chew gum or use a saliva substitute.

 While taking this medicine you should tell your doctor if you become pregnant or plan to become pregnant or if you are breast-feeding an infant.

If you miss a dose of this medicine, take it as soon as possible. But, if it is almost time for your next dose, skip the missed dose and go back to your regular dose. DO NOT take a double dose.

DO NOT keep or use outdated medicine. Keep this medicine at room temperature, in its original container and out of the reach of children.

POSSIBLE SIDE EFFECTS:

 Be sure to tell your doctor if the following occur: nausea, diarrhea, nervousness or confusion, irregular heartbeat or pulse, fainting spells, difficulty getting to sleep or urinating, severe drowsiness, troubled breathing, high fever or hallucinations.

MAXAQUIN

THIS MEDICATION IS USED:

To treat infections.

PROPER USE OF THIS MEDICATION:

 This medication can be taken with or without regards to food.

If stomach upsets occurs, take it with food.

 DO NOT take antacids or iron supplements within 2 hours of taking this medication.

SPECIAL INSTRUCTIONS:

 The recommended length of treatment is 10-14 days. You should take all the medication unless otherwise instructed by your doctor.

 It is recommended that you drink lots of fluids while you are taking this medication.

 You may experience dizziness, blurred vision or drowsiness from this medicine. If you do, be careful driving or performing hazardous tasks.

 This medicine may make your skin more sensitive to sunlight or sunlamps. Ask your pharmacist about a suitable sunblock product (of at least SPF 15) to minimize problems during exposure.

If you miss a dose of this medicine, take it as soon as possible. But, if it is almost time for your next dose, take the missed dose, space the next dose 10-12 hours apart and then go back to your regular dosing schedule. DO NOT take a double dose.

DO NOT keep or use outdated medication. Keep all medication out of the reach of children.

POSSIBLE SIDE EFFECTS:

 Be sure to tell your doctor if the following occur: skin rash, nausea or vomiting, headache, diarrhea, blurred vision, excessive dizziness or drowsiness, stomach pain or dry mouth.

IMODIUM (RX), LOPERAMIDE

THIS MEDICATION IS USED:

To treat diarrhea.

PROPER USE OF THIS MEDICATION:

 Take this medicine with a glass of water. If it upsets your stomach you may take it with food.

SPECIAL INSTRUCTIONS:

If your diarrhea does not stop after a few days or if you develop a high fever, call your doctor.

 You may experience dizziness or drowsiness from this medicine. If you do, be careful driving or performing hazardous tasks.

 Alcoholic beverages can increase drowsiness.

If your mouth becomes dry, you may suck on hard candy, chew gum or use a saliva substitute.

 You should drink extra fluids each day to help replace the fluid your body has lost due to the diarrhea.

If you miss a dose of this medicine, take it as soon as possible. If it is almost time for your next dose, skip the missed dose and go back to your regular dose. DO NOT take a double dose.

DO NOT keep or use outdated medication. Keep all medication out of the reach of children.

POSSIBLE SIDE EFFECTS:

 Be sure to tell your doctor if the following occur: nausea or vomiting, shallow breathing, unusual excitement or depression or prolonged fever.

SELDANE D

THIS MEDICATION IS USED:

To relieve the runny nose, watery eyes, sneezing and stuffiness of colds and hay fever. It may also be used for allergic reactions.

PROPER USE OF THIS MEDICATION:

 This medicine should be swallowed whole. It may be taken with or without food.

If it upsets your stomach take it with food.

SPECIAL INSTRUCTIONS:

If your mouth becomes dry, you may suck on hard candy, chew gum or use a saliva substitute.

It is important that you take this medicine exactly as your doctor has instructed. Take this only as needed and DO NOT take more doses than prescribed by your doctor.

 DO NOT take nonprescription cough/cold or diet products without asking your doctor or pharmacist.

You should talk with your doctor before taking the following prescription medications: erythromycin derivatives, ketoconazole (Nizoral), or itraconazole (Sporanox).

 Tell your doctor if you are pregnant, plan to become pregnant or are breastfeeding.

If you miss a dose of this medicine, take it as soon as possible. But, if it is almost time for your next dose, skip the missed dose and go back to your regular dosing schedule. DO NOT take a double dose.

DO NOT keep or use outdated medication. Keep all medication out of the reach of children.

POSSIBLE SIDE EFFECTS:

 Be sure to tell your doctor if the following occur: thickening of the bronchial secretions, headache, dry mouth, blurred vision, drowsiness, increased appetite, nervousness, dizziness, nausea or upset stomach, chest pain or irregular heartbeat.

FLOXIN

THIS MEDICATION IS USED:

To treat infections.

PROPER USE OF THIS MEDICATION:

 This medication should be taken on an empty stomach, either one hour before or two hours after a meal.

 DO NOT take antacids or iron supplements within 2 hours of taking this medication.

SPECIAL INSTRUCTIONS:

 The recommended length of treatment is 7-10 days. You should take all the medication unless otherwise instructed by your doctor.

 It is recommended that you drink lots of fluids while you are taking this medication.

 You may experience dizziness, blurred vision or drowsiness from this medicine. If you do, be careful driving or performing hazardous tasks.

 This medicine may make your skin more sensitive to sunlight or sunlamps. Ask your pharmacist about a suitable sunblock product (of at least SPF 15) to minimize problems during exposure.

Stop this medicine at the first sign of a skin rash or other allergic reaction and tell your doctor.

If you miss a dose of this medicine, take it as soon as possible. But, if it is almost time for your next dose, skip the missed dose and go back to your regular dosing schedule. DO NOT take a double dose.

DO NOT keep or use outdated medication. Keep all medication out of the reach of children.

POSSIBLE SIDE EFFECTS:

 Be sure to tell your doctor if the following occur: skin rash, nausea or vomiting, headache, diarrhea, blurred vision, dizziness or drowsiness, stomach pain or dry mouth.

METHOTREXATE, RHEUMATREX

THIS MEDICINE IS USED:

To treat rheumatoid arthritis, psoriasis and other conditions determined by your doctor.

PROPER USE OF THIS MEDICATION:

 This medication can be taken with or without food. It is best to drink a lot of fluids with each dose and throughout the day (6-8 glassfuls).

 Some treatment schedules are unusual, i.e. 2-6 tablets once a WEEK. Be sure you understand and follow your doctor's instructions exactly. Taking more than the prescribed dose can cause very serious side effects.

SPECIAL INSTRUCTIONS:

 DO NOT drink alcoholic beverages while taking this medication. Alcohol can increase side effects.

 DO NOT take nonprescription pain medications without asking your doctor or pharmacist. Aspirin and ibuprofen can increase side effects.

 This medicine may make your skin more sensitive to sunlight and sunlamps. Ask your pharmacist about a suitable sunblock product (of at least SPF 15) to minimize problems during exposure.

 While this medication exerts its needed actions, it can cause annoying side effects. Among these are nausea and vomiting. If you become nauseated, DO NOT stop taking the medicine without first checking with your doctor. If you vomit shortly after taking a dose, or, if vomiting continues check with your doctor right away.

This medicine may lower your resistance to infections. If you feel you are coming down with a cold or the flu, or, any other infection, call your doctor right away.

Be sure you keep all appointments for lab tests ordered by your doctor.

If you forgot to take the scheduled dose of this medicine, call your doctor right away for instructions on what to do. You should NOT take a double dose without asking your doctor first.

This medication is known to cause birth defects and fetal death. Pregnancy should be avoided if it is taken by either partner and for several months after it is discontinued.

DO NOT keep or use outdated medication. Keep this medication in its original container at room temperature and out of the reach of children.

POSSIBLE SIDE EFFECTS:

Be sure to tell your doctor right away if the following occur: unusual bleeding or bruising; sores or bleeding on the inside of your mouth or on your gums; severe, persistent vomiting or diarrhea, especially if blood is present or the stools are black and tarry looking; painful or difficult urination or blood in the urine; stomach pain; or, reddening or red spots on your skin.

TORADOL

THIS MEDICATION IS USED:

For the relief of pain.

PROPER USE OF THIS MEDICATION:

Take this medicine with a glass of water. If it upsets your stomach you may take it with food.

SPECIAL INSTRUCTIONS:

DO NOT take nonprescription ibuprofen, aspirin or acetaminophen products while taking this drug without checking with your doctor or pharmacist.

You may experience dizziness, blurred vision or drowsiness from this medicine. If you do, be careful driving or performing hazardous tasks.

If you continue to experience stomach upset while taking this medicine, you should tell your doctor.

If you miss a dose of this medicine, take it as soon as possible. But, if it is almost time for your next dose, skip the missed dose and take your regular dose. DO NOT take a double dose.

DO NOT keep or use outdated medicine. Keep this medicine at room temperature, in its original container and out of the reach of children.

POSSIBLE SIDE EFFECTS:

Be sure to tell your doctor if any of the following occur: skin rash, ringing or buzzing in the ears, changed vision, stomach pain or nausea, persistent sore throat or fever, black, tarry or bloody stools, unusual weight gain or edema in the extremities or difficulty in breathing.

NICOTINE PATCH
Habitrol Transdermal, Nicoderm Transdermal, Nicotrol Transdermal, Prostep Transdermal

THIS MEDICATION IS USED:

As a temporary aid to help stop smoking.

PROPER USE OF THIS MEDICATION:

 Apply the patch to a clean, dry, non-hairy area of skin on your upper body or upper outer part of your arm. Avoid skin that is irritated.

Remove the protective liner and press the patch firmly on your skin, making sure that the edges stick well.

When removing the old patch, fold it in half with the sticky side together. Place it in the pouch that the new patch was removed from, wrap this in newspaper and discard in the trash.

 Wash your hands when finished applying or discarding the patch.

 Apply the new patch at approximately the same time every day. Always remember to rotate the site of application.

If the patch falls off, put on a new patch and remove it at your regular time in order to stay on schedule.

Water WILL NOT harm the patch you are wearing. You can bathe, shower or swim while wearing these patches.

It is not unusual for the skin to tingle, itch or burn when a patch is first applied. This is normal and should go away within an hour. If it continues, contact your doctor.

 It is not unusual for the skin to be red or a darker color after removing a patch. This SHOULD NOT last for more than a day. If it does or the area becomes inflamed, contact your doctor.

SPECIAL INSTRUCTIONS:

This product WILL NOT cure your smoking habit. The best method is to internalize your desire to be a nonsmoker. This product will help offset your cravings for nicotine while quitting.

This product is intended to be an aid to participation in a behavioral modification program. There are a number of "quitters" programs available, ask your doctor or pharmacist for information about them.

You must be committed to quit smoking or this product WILL NOT work.

 For this product to work you must use it exactly as directed. DO NOT smoke while you are using it as this can lead to side effects.

Instructions for each brand of patch are similar, but slightly different. Read them carefully and follow the directions. If you have any questions, ask your doctor or pharmacist.

The used patches must be discarded correctly to prevent poisoning in children and pets.

If you notice any worrisome symptoms or problems, take off the patch and call your doctor at once.

If there is a chance that pregnancy has occurred, stop smoking and DO NOT use these patches until you have talked to your doctor.

If you miss a dose, apply at once and return to your regular schedule. DO NOT double a dose.

Keep each patch in its protective pouch at room temperature until you are ready to use it. DO NOT expose the patches to excessive heat.

DO NOT keep or use outdated medication. Keep all medication out of the reach of children.

POSSIBLE SIDE EFFECTS:

 Be sure to tell your doctor if the following occur: persistent headache, dizziness, upset stomach, nausea or vomiting, rapid heart beat, blurred vision, difficulty in hearing, or mental confusion.

CORTICOSTEROID (INTRANASAL SPRAY)
Beconase AQ, Nasalide, Vancenase AQ

THIS MEDICATION IS USED:

In the nose to relieve or prevent the discomfort of hay fever and other nasal problems.

PROPER USE OF THIS MEDICATION:

 Remove the dust cap and safety clip and shake the bottle well before using it.

Gently blow your nose to clear the nostrils just before using this medicine.

 Close one nostril with your finger, tilt head slightly forward and carefully insert the nasal applicator into the open nostril.

Press downward firmly using your forefinger and middle finger, while using your thumb on the base for support.

Breathe gently inward through the nostril and breathe out through the mouth.

Repeat in other nostril.

Replace the dust cap and safety clip after use.

SPECIAL INSTRUCTIONS:

 To help prevent contamination from nasal secretions, rinse the applicator in warm water after each use.

 Instructions for each brand of nasal spray are similar, but slightly different. Read them carefully and follow the directions. If you have any questions, ask your doctor or pharmacist.

 Proper control of your condition requires you to use this medicine as instructed at the same time every day, DO NOT skip a dose nor stop using the medicine without asking your doctor.

It is important that you continue using this medicine as your doctor has instructed. It may take several days before improvement is noticed.

For the first 2-3 days, if you have excessive nasal congestion, you may use a decongestant nasal spray just prior to using this medication.

If you miss a dose of this medicine, use it as soon as possible. But, if it is almost time for your next dose, skip the missed dose and go back to your regular dose. DO NOT use a double dose.

DO NOT keep or use outdated medicine. Keep this medicine at room temperature, in its original container and out of the reach of children.

POSSIBLE SIDE EFFECTS:

 Be sure to tell your doctor if the following occur: continued nasal irritation, excessive sneezing, bloody discharge from the nose, persistent sore throat, swelling of the face, hands or feet, skin rash, difficulty in breathing or muscle cramps or pain.

PROSCAR

THIS MEDICATION IS USED:

To treat the symptoms of a condition referred to as benign prostatic hyperplasia (BPH).

PROPER USE OF THIS MEDICATION:

 This medication should be taken with a glass of water and it can be taken with or without food.

SPECIAL INSTRUCTIONS:

 Proper control of your condition requires you to take this medicine as instructed at the same time every day, DO NOT skip a dose nor stop taking the medicine without asking your doctor.

It may take at least 6 months of treatment to determine if you will respond to Proscar.

 Crushed Proscar tablets SHOULD NOT be handled by a woman who is pregnant or who may become pregnant because of the potential risk to a male fetus. Also, when the patient's sexual partner is or may become pregnant, the patient should avoid exposure of his partner to semen.

The amount of ejaculate may be decreased during treatment with Proscar. This decrease does not interfere with normal sexual function.

If you miss a dose of this medicine, take it as soon as possible. But, if it is almost time for your next dose, skip the missed dose and go back to your regular dose. DO NOT take a double dose.

DO NOT keep or use outdated medicine. Keep this medicine at room temperature, in its original container and out of the reach of children.

POSSIBLE SIDE EFFECTS:

 Be sure to tell your doctor if the following occur: impotence or a loss of sexual drive.

DILACOR XR

THIS MEDICATION IS USED:

 To treat high blood pressure.

PROPER USE OF THIS MEDICATION:

 Unless your doctor has told you differently, this medicine should be taken on an empty stomach with a glass of water at least 1 hour before or 2 hours after a meal.

 This is a controlled release capsule, which should be swallowed whole. DO NOT open, chew, or crush this medicine.

SPECIAL INSTRUCTIONS:

 This medicine may cause lightheadedness. Sit or lie down at the first signs. Avoid sudden changes in posture. Be careful going up and down stairs. Be careful driving or performing hazardous tasks.

The use of alcohol while taking this medicine may increase the chance of dizziness.

 Proper control of your condition requires you to take this medicine as instructed at the same time every day, DO NOT skip a dose nor stop taking the medicine without asking your doctor.

Since this medicine does not cure but helps to control your condition, you should continue to take it even if you are feeling well.

 DO NOT take nonprescription cough/cold or diet products without asking your doctor or pharmacist.

If you miss a dose of this medicine, take it as soon as possible. But, if it is almost time for your next dose, skip the missed dose and go back to your regular dose. DO NOT take a double dose.

DO NOT keep or use outdated medicine. Keep this medicine at room temperature, in its original container and out of the reach of children.

POSSIBLE SIDE EFFECTS:

 Be sure to tell your doctor if the following occur: headache, nausea, swelling of the extremities, unusually slow heartbeat, chest pain, unusual tiredness or difficult breathing.

ATROVENT INHALER

THIS MEDICATION IS USED:

To treat the symptoms of bronchial asthma, chronic bronchitis and emphysema.

PROPER USE OF THIS MEDICATION:

BE SURE the canister is properly inserted into the inhaler unit.

 REMOVE dust cap and SHAKE the can WELL.

Hold the inhaler with the nozzle down.

Unless your doctor has told you otherwise, exhale fully and place mouthpiece into your mouth with your lips closed around it and your tongue flat.

As you take a deep breath, squeeze the can and mouthpiece together at exactly the same time.

Continue taking a deep breath and hold it for as long as comfortable.

Exhale slowly, keeping your lips nearly closed.

Desired relief may not be immediate. Be sure to wait the prescribed time before inhaling a second dose.

SPECIAL INSTRUCTIONS:

 KEEP THE MOUTHPIECE CLEAN. At least once daily, wash the mouthpiece with soap and hot water. Rinse thoroughly and allow to dry.

The contents of the can are under pressure. DO NOT puncture or throw it into an incinerator.

When not using the inhaler, store it with the dust cap on the mouthpiece. This will prevent dirt and dust from getting into the mouthpiece.

Proper control of your condition requires you to use this medicine as instructed at the same time every day, DO NOT skip a dose nor stop using the medicine without asking your doctor.

It is important that you continue using this medicine as your doctor has instructed.

 DO NOT spray this medication in the eyes.

If you are using other aerosol medications, wait at least 5 minutes before using each medication to achieve the best results. If the other medication is a bronchodilator, this should be used first. If the other medication is a corticosteroid, then Atrovent should be used first. If you have any questions, ask your doctor or pharmacist.

 DO NOT take nonprescription cough/cold, hay fever or sleep aid products without asking your doctor or pharmacist.

If you miss a dose of this medicine, use it as soon as possible. But, if it is almost time for your next dose, skip the missed dose and go back to your regular dose. DO NOT take a double dose.

DO NOT keep or use outdated medicine. Keep this medicine at room temperature, in its original container and out of the reach of children.

POSSIBLE SIDE EFFECTS:

 Be sure to tell your doctor if the following occur: eye pain or blurred vision, dryness of mouth, persistent cough, nausea, dizziness, severe headache, nervousness, or skin rash.

NOLVADEX

THIS MEDICATION IS USED:

To treat breast cancer and other conditions as determined by your doctor.

PROPER USE OF THIS MEDICINE:

 Take this medicine with a glass of water. If it upsets your stomach you may take it with food.

SPECIAL INSTRUCTIONS:

It is important that you take this medicine exactly as your doctor has instructed.

 Proper control of your condition requires you to take this medicine as instructed at the same time every day, DO NOT skip a dose nor stop taking the medicine without asking your doctor.

 DO NOT take this medication if you are pregnant and DO NOT become pregnant while taking it.

If there is a chance that pregnancy has occurred call your doctor right away.

If you miss a dose of this medicine, take it as soon as possible. But, if it is almost time for your next dose, skip the missed dose and go back to your regular dose. DO NOT take a double dose.

DO NOT keep or use outdated medicine. Keep this medicine at room temperature, in its original container and out of the reach of children.

POSSIBLE SIDE EFFECTS:

 Be sure to tell your doctor if the following occur: hot flashes, dizziness or headache, bone pain, pain or swelling of legs, blurred vision, muscle weakness or pain, confusion, shortness of breath, loss of taste or appetite, fatigue, nausea or vomiting or menstrual irregularities.

PARLODEL

THIS MEDICATION IS USED:

To treat Parkinson's disease. It is also used to treat hormonal problems and other conditions as determined by your doctor.

PROPER USE OF THIS MEDICATION:

Take this medication with food and a glass of water to help avoid upsetting your stomach.

SPECIAL INSTRUCTIONS:

You may experience dizziness, blurred vision or drowsiness from this medicine. If you do, be careful driving or performing hazardous tasks.

Alcoholic beverages can increase the drowsiness.

This medicine may cause lightheadedness. Sit or lie down at the first signs. Avoid sudden changes in posture. Be careful going up and down stairs.

Proper control of your condition requires you to take this medicine as instructed at the same time every day, DO NOT skip a dose nor stop taking the medicine without asking your doctor.

DO NOT change the amount of medicine taken without consulting your doctor.

If your mouth becomes dry, you may suck on hard candy, chew gum or use a saliva substitute.

If you miss a dose of this medicine, take it as soon as possible. But, if it is almost time for your next dose, skip the missed dose and go back to your regular dose. DO NOT take a double dose.

DO NOT keep or use outdated medicine. Keep this medicine at room temperature, in its original container and out of the reach of children.

POSSIBLE SIDE EFFECTS:

Be sure to tell your doctor if the following occur: severe headache, excessive dizziness or drowsiness, blurred vision, rapid heartbeat, confusion, nausea, difficulty in urination, numbness in the hands or feet or persistent watery nasal discharge.

PERMAX

THIS MEDICATION IS USED:

To treat Parkinson's Disease.

PROPER USE OF THIS MEDICATION:

Take this medicine with a glass of water. If it upsets your stomach you may take it with food.

SPECIAL INSTRUCTIONS:

You may experience dizziness, blurred vision or drowsiness from this medicine. If you do, be careful driving or performing hazardous tasks.

Alcoholic beverages can increase the drowsiness.

This medicine may cause lightheadedness. Sit or lie down at the first signs. Avoid sudden changes in posture. Be careful going up and down stairs.

Proper control of your condition requires you to take this medicine as instructed at the same time every day, DO NOT skip a dose nor stop taking the medicine without asking your doctor.

DO NOT change the amount of medicine taken without consulting your doctor.

While taking this medicine you should tell your doctor if you become pregnant or plan to become pregnant or if you are breast-feeding an infant.

If your mouth becomes dry, you may suck on hard candy, chew gum or use a saliva substitute.

If you miss a dose of this medicine, take it as soon as possible. But, if it is almost time for your next dose, skip the missed dose and go back to your regular dose. DO NOT take a double dose.

DO NOT keep or use outdated medicine. Keep this medicine at room temperature, in its original container and out of the reach of children.

POSSIBLE SIDE EFFECTS:

 Be sure to tell your doctor if the following occur: severe headache, excessive dizziness or drowsiness, blurred vision, rapid heartbeat, confusion, nausea, difficulty in urination, numbness in the hands or feet, runny nose, constipation or skin rash.

PENETREX

THIS MEDICATION IS USED:

To treat infections.

PROPER USE OF THIS MEDICATION:

 This medication should be taken on an empty stomach, either one hour before or two hours after a meal.

 DO NOT take antacids, iron or zinc supplements or bismuth subsalicylate products 8 hours before or 2 hours after taking this medication.

SPECIAL INSTRUCTIONS:

 The recommended length of treatment is 7-10 days. You should take all the medication unless otherwise instructed by your doctor.

 It is recommended that you drink lots of fluids while you are taking this medication.

 You may experience dizziness, blurred vision or drowsiness from this medicine. If you do, be careful driving or performing hazardous tasks.

 This medicine may make your skin more sensitive to sunlight or sunlamps. Ask your pharmacist about a suitable sunblock product (of at least SPF 15) to minimize problems during exposure.

Stop this medicine if you develop a skin rash or other allergic reaction and tell your doctor.

Be careful taking products containing caffeine while on this medicine, as there may be increased caffeine-related stimulation.

If you miss a dose of this medicine, take it as soon as possible. But, if it is almost time for your next dose, skip the missed dose and go back to your regular dosing schedule.

DO NOT take a double dose.

DO NOT keep or use outdated medicine. Keep this medicine at room temperature, in its original container and out of the reach of children.

POSSIBLE SIDE EFFECTS:

 Be sure to tell your doctor if the following occur: skin rash, nausea or vomiting, headache, diarrhea, blurred vision, dizziness or drowsiness, stomach pain or dry mouth.

NIZORAL ORAL
Nizoral Tablet

THIS MEDICATION IS USED:

To treat fungal infections and other conditions as determined by your doctor.

PROPER USE OF THIS MEDICATION:

 Take this medicine with a glass of water. If it upsets your stomach you may take it with food.

SPECIAL INSTRUCTIONS:

 Long term therapy is needed (possibly 3 months or longer). It is important to take the full length of treatment unless otherwise instructed by your doctor.

DO NOT change the amount of medicine taken nor stop taking it without consulting your doctor.

 You may experience dizziness, blurred vision or drowsiness from this medicine. If you do, be careful driving or performing hazardous tasks.

Alcoholic beverages can increase the drowsiness.

 You should talk with your doctor before taking the following prescription medications: astemizole (Hismanal) and terfenadine (Seldane, Seldane-D).

If you miss a dose of this medicine, take it as soon as possible. But, if it is almost time for your next dose, space the missed dose and the next dose 10-12 hours apart. Then go back to your regular schedule. DO NOT take a double dose.

DO NOT keep or use outdated medicine. Keep this medicine at room temperature, in its original container and out of the reach of children.

POSSIBLE SIDE EFFECTS:

 Be sure to tell your doctor if the following occur: dizziness, drowsiness or confusion, nausea or vomiting, stomach pain, severe headache, diarrhea, yellowing of the skin or eyes, loss of appetite or dark or amber colored urine.

SPORANOX

THIS MEDICATION IS USED:

To treat fungal infections.

PROPER USE OF THIS MEDICATION:

 To maximize absorption and to reduce the chance of stomach upset, this medicine SHOULD be taken with food.

SPECIAL INSTRUCTIONS:

 Long term therapy is needed (possibly 3 months or longer). It is important to take the full length of treatment unless otherwise instructed by your doctor.

DO NOT change the amount of medicine taken nor stop taking it without consulting your doctor.

 You may experience dizziness, blurred vision or drowsiness from this medicine. If you do, be careful driving or performing hazardous tasks.

Alcoholic beverages can increase the drowsiness.

 You should talk with your doctor before taking the following prescription medications: astemizole (Hismanal) and terfenadine (Seldane, Seldane-D).

If you miss a dose of this medicine, take it as soon as possible. But, if it is almost time for your next dose, space the missed dose and the next dose 10-12 hours apart. Then go back to your regular schedule. DO NOT take a double dose.

DO NOT keep or use outdated medicine. Keep this medicine at room temperature, in its original container and out of the reach of children.

POSSIBLE SIDE EFFECTS:

Be sure to tell your doctor if the following occur: dizziness, drowsiness or confusion, nausea or vomiting, stomach pain, severe headache, diarrhea, yellowing of the skin or eyes, loss of appetite or dark or amber colored urine.

EXPECTORANT & NARCOTIC ANTITUSSIVE

Codiclear DH, Dilaudid Liquid, Entuss, Glycerol C, Guiatuss AC, Guiatussin w/Codeine, Hycotuss, Iodinated Glycerol w/Codeine, Iophen C, Iotuss, Robitussin AC, Tussi-Organidin, Tussi-R-Gen

THIS MEDICATION IS USED:

For the symptomatic relief of coughs.

PROPER USE OF THIS MEDICATION:

 Take this medicine with a glass of water. If it upsets your stomach you may take it with food.

If you are taking the liquid form, there are special measuring devices available to measure your dose, ask your pharmacist if you want one.

SPECIAL INSTRUCTIONS:

 You may experience dizziness, blurred vision or drowsiness from this medicine. If you do, be careful driving or performing hazardous tasks.

Alcoholic beverages can increase the drowsiness.

If your mouth becomes dry, you may suck on hard candy, chew gum or use a saliva substitute.

 If taken for a few days, you may experience some constipation. You should increase the amount of bulk in your diet (bran, psyllium, and fresh fruits) and drink lots of fluids.

 DO NOT take nonprescription cough/cold products without asking your doctor or pharmacist.

If you miss a dose of this medicine, take it as soon as possible. But, if it is almost time for your next dose, skip the missed dose and go back to your regular dosing schedule. DO NOT take a double dose.

DO NOT keep or use outdated medicine. Keep this medicine at room temperature, in its original container and out of the reach of children.

POSSIBLE SIDE EFFECTS:

 Be sure to tell your doctor if the following occur: drowsiness, dizziness or lightheadedness, nausea or vomiting, heartburn or indigestion, difficult breathing, unusual heartbeat, sweating, excitement or skin rash.

EXPECTORANT & NONNARCOTIC ANTITUSSIVE

Glycerol DM, Humibid DM LA, Humibid DM Sprinkle,
Iodinated Glycerol DM, Iophen DM, Iotuss DM,
Tussi-Organidin DM, Tussi-R-Gen DM

THIS MEDICATION IS USED:

For the symptomatic relief of coughs.

PROPER USE OF THIS MEDICATION:

 Take this medicine with a glass of water. If it upsets your stomach you may take it with food.

If you are taking the liquid form, there are special measuring devices available to measure your dose, ask your pharmacist if you want one.

 The controlled release forms should be swallowed whole, NOT crushed or chewed.

SPECIAL INSTRUCTIONS:

 You may experience dizziness, blurred vision or drowsiness from this medicine. If you do, be careful driving or performing hazardous tasks.

Alcoholic beverages can increase the drowsiness.

If your mouth becomes dry, you may suck on hard candy, chew gum or use a saliva substitute.

 DO NOT take nonprescription cough/cold products without asking your doctor or pharmacist.

It is recommended that you drink lots of fluids while taking this medication.

If you miss a dose of this medicine, take it as soon as possible. But, if it is almost time for your next dose, skip the missed dose and go back to your regular dosing schedule. DO NOT take a double dose.

DO NOT keep or use outdated medicine. Keep this medicine at room temperature, in its original container and out of the reach of children.

POSSIBLE SIDE EFFECTS:

 Be sure to tell your doctor if the following occur: drowsiness, dizziness or lightheadedness, nausea or vomiting, or heartburn or indigestion.

DECONGESTANT & EXPECTORANT & NARCOTIC ANTITUSSIVE

Detussin Exp, Dihistine, Endal Liquid, Entuss D Tablet, Guiatuss DAC, Guiatussin DAC, Naldecon CX, Nucofed Liquid, Nucofed Pediatric, Phenhist, Robitussin DAC, Triaminic w/Codeine, Tussafin, Vanex

THIS MEDICATION IS USED:

To relieve the symptoms of nasal stuffiness and coughs.

PROPER USE OF THIS MEDICATION:

Take this medicine with a glass of water. If it upsets your stomach you may take it with food.

If you are taking the liquid form, there are special measuring devices available to measure your dose, ask your pharmacist if you want one.

SPECIAL INSTRUCTIONS:

You may experience dizziness, blurred vision or drowsiness from this medicine. If you do, be careful driving or performing hazardous tasks.

Alcoholic beverages can increase the drowsiness.

If your mouth becomes dry, you may suck on hard candy, chew gum or use a saliva substitute.

If taken for a few days, you may experience some constipation. You should increase the amount of bulk in your diet (bran, psyllium, and fresh fruits) and drink lots of fluids.

DO NOT take nonprescription cough/cold or diet products without asking your doctor or pharmacist.

If you miss a dose of this medicine, take it as soon as possible. But, if it is almost time for your next dose, skip the missed dose and go back to your regular dosing schedule. DO NOT take a double dose.

DO NOT keep or use outdated medicine. Keep this medicine at room temperature, in its original container and out of the reach of children.

POSSIBLE SIDE EFFECTS:

Be sure to tell your doctor if the following occur: persistent headache, restlessness, nausea or vomiting, heartburn or indigestion, difficulty in breathing or sleeping, unusual heartbeat, sweating, excitement or skin rash.

DECONGESTANT & EXPECTORANT & NONNARCOTIC ANTITUSSIVE

Antatuss, Rutuss Exp

THIS MEDICATION IS USED:

To relieve the symptoms of nasal stuffiness and coughs.

PROPER USE OF THIS MEDICATION:

 Take this medicine with a glass of water. If it upsets your stomach you may take it with food.

If you are taking the liquid form, there are special measuring devices available to measure your dose, ask your pharmacist if you want one.

SPECIAL INSTRUCTIONS:

 You may experience dizziness, blurred vision or drowsiness from this medicine. If you do, be careful driving or performing hazardous tasks.

Alcoholic beverages can increase the drowsiness.

If your mouth becomes dry, you may suck on hard candy, chew gum or use a saliva substitute.

 It is recommended that you drink lots of fluids while taking this medication.

 DO NOT take nonprescription cough/cold or diet products without asking your doctor or pharmacist.

If you miss a dose of this medicine, take it as soon as possible. But, if it is almost time for your next dose, skip the missed dose and go back to your regular dosing schedule. DO NOT take a double dose.

DO NOT keep or use outdated medicine. Keep this medicine at room temperature, in its original container and out of the reach of children.

POSSIBLE SIDE EFFECTS:

 Be sure to tell you doctor if the following occur: persistent headache, restlessness, nausea or vomiting, heartburn or indigestion, difficulty in sleeping, unusual heartbeat, sweating, excitement or skin rash.

ANTIHISTAMINE & NARCOTIC ANTITUSSIVE
Phenergan w/Codeine, Tussionex

THIS MEDICATION IS USED:

To relieve the runny nose, watery eyes, coughing and sneezing of colds and hay fever.

PROPER USE OF THIS MEDICATION:

 Take this medicine with a glass of water, if it upsets your stomach you may take it with food.

Some of the liquid forms require the contents to be shaken well just before measuring the dose.

 There are special measuring devices available, ask your pharmacist if you want one.

SPECIAL INSTRUCTIONS:

 You may experience dizziness, blurred vision or drowsiness from this medicine. If you do, be careful driving or performing hazardous tasks.

Alcoholic beverages can increase the drowsiness.

If your mouth becomes dry, you may suck on hard candy, chew gum or use a saliva substitute.

 If taken for a few days, you may experience some constipation. You should increase the amount of bulk in your diet (bran, psyllium, and fresh fruits) and drink lots of fluids.

 This medicine may make your skin more sensitive to sunlight or sunlamps. Ask your pharmacist about a suitable sunblock product (of at least SPF 15) to minimize problems during exposure.

 DO NOT take nonprescription cough/cold, hay fever or sleep aid products without asking your doctor or pharmacist.

If you miss a dose of this medicine, take it as soon as possible. But, if it is almost time for your next dose, skip the

missed dose and go back to your regular dose. DO NOT take a double dose.

DO NOT keep or use outdated medicine. Keep this medicine at room temperature, in its original container and out of the reach of children.

POSSIBLE SIDE EFFECTS:

Be sure to tell your doctor if the following occur: drowsiness, blurred vision, dry mouth, headache, mental confusion, loss of appetite, difficulty in breathing, unusual heartbeat, sweating, excitement or skin rash.

DECONGESTANT & NARCOTIC ANTITUSSIVE

Codamine, Detussin, Entuss D Liquid, Hycomine, Nucofed Capsule, Phenylpropanolamine w/Hydrocodone, Tussgen

THIS MEDICATION IS USED:

To treat the symptoms of nasal stuffiness and coughs due to colds.

PROPER USE OF THIS MEDICATION:

Take this medicine with a glass of water. If it upsets your stomach you may take it with food.

If you are taking the liquid form, there are special measuring devices available to measure your dose, ask your pharmacist if you want one.

SPECIAL INSTRUCTIONS:

You may experience dizziness, blurred vision or drowsiness from this medicine. If you do, be careful driving or performing hazardous tasks.

Alcoholic beverages can increase the drowsiness.

If your mouth becomes dry, you may suck on hard candy, chew gum or use a saliva substitute.

If taken for a few days, you may experience some constipation. You should increase the amount of bulk in your diet (bran, psyllium, and fresh fruits) and drink lots of fluids.

DO NOT take nonprescription cough/cold or diet products without asking your doctor or pharmacist.

If you miss a dose of this medicine, take it as soon as possible. But, if it is almost time for your next dose, skip the missed dose and go back to your regular dosing schedule. DO NOT take a double dose.

DO NOT keep or use outdated medicine. Keep this medicine at room temperature, in its original container and out of the reach of children.

POSSIBLE SIDE EFFECTS:

 Be sure to tell your doctor if the following occur: persistent headache, restlessness, nausea or vomiting, heartburn or indigestion, difficulty in breathing or sleeping, unusual heartbeat, sweating, excitement or skin rash.

ANTIHISTAMINE & NONNARCOTIC ANTITUSSIVE

Phenergan DM, Promethazine DM

THIS MEDICATION IS USED:

To relieve the runny nose, watery eyes, coughing and sneezing of colds and hay fever.

PROPER USE OF THIS MEDICATION:

Take this medicine with a glass of water. If it upsets your stomach you may take it with food.

The controlled release forms should be swallowed whole, NOT crushed or chewed.

If you are taking the liquid form, there are special measuring devices available to measure your dose, ask your pharmacist if you want one.

SPECIAL INSTRUCTIONS:

You may experience dizziness, blurred vision or drowsiness from this medicine. If you do, be careful driving or performing hazardous tasks.

Alcoholic beverages can increase the drowsiness.

If your mouth becomes dry, you may suck on hard candy, chew gum or use a saliva substitute.

It is recommended that you drink lots of fluids while taking this medication.

This medicine may make your skin more sensitive to sunlight or sunlamps. Ask your pharmacist about a suitable sunblock product (of at least SPF 15) to minimize problems during exposure.

DO NOT take nonprescription cough/cold, hay fever or sleep aid products without asking your doctor or pharmacist.

If you miss a dose of this medicine, take it as soon as possible. But, if it is almost time for your next dose, skip the

missed dose and go back to your regular dose. DO NOT take a double dose.

DO NOT keep or use outdated medicine. Keep this medicine at room temperature, in its original container and out of the reach of children.

POSSIBLE SIDE EFFECTS:

 Be sure to tell your doctor if the following occur: drowsiness, blurred vision, dry mouth, headache, mental confusion, nausea or vomiting, or heartburn or indigestion.

ZITHROMAX

THIS MEDICATION IS USED:

To treat infections.

PROPER USE OF THIS MEDICATION:

 Unless your doctor has told you differently, this medicine should be taken on an empty stomach with a glass of water at least 1 hour before or 2 hours after a meal.

 DO NOT take antacids within 2 hours of taking this medicine.

SPECIAL INSTRUCTIONS:

 The recommended length of treatment is 5 days. You should take all the medication unless otherwise instructed by your doctor.

 If you experience diarrhea while taking this medicine, DO NOT take any antidiarrheal medicine without first asking your doctor or pharmacist.

If you miss a dose, take the missed dose as soon as possible. But if it is almost time for your next dose, space the missed dose and the next dose 10-12 hours apart. Then go back to your regular dosing schedule.

DO NOT keep or use outdated medicine. Keep this medicine at room temperature, in its original container and out of the reach of children.

POSSIBLE SIDE EFFECTS:

 Be sure to tell your doctor if the following occur: prolonged or severe nausea, vomiting or diarrhea, abdominal pain or irregular heartbeat.

INDEX

INDEX

INDEX

INDEX

INDEX

INDEX

INDEX

INDEX

INDEX

INDEX

INDEX